Recent Advances in

Surgery

Recent Advances in Surgery 23
Edited by C. D. Johnson & I. Taylor

ISBN 0-443-064423
ISSN 0143 8395

NUMBER
24

Recent Advances in

Surgery

Edited by

I. Taylor MD ChM FRCS

David Patey Professor of Surgery, Royal Free and University College London
Medical School, University College London, London, UK

C. D. Johnson MChir FRCS

Reader and Consultant Surgeon, University Surgical Unit, Southampton
General Hospital, Southampton, UK

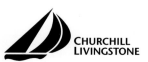
CHURCHILL
LIVINGSTONE

EDINBURGH LONDON NEW YORK PHILADELPHIA St LOUIS SYDNEY TORONTO 2001

CHURCHILL LIVINGSTONE
An imprint of Harcourt Publishers Limited

© Harcourt Publishers Limited 2001

First published 2001

ISBN 0-443-070660

ISSN 0143 8395

British Library Cataloguing in Publication Data
A catalogue record for this book is available from the British Library

Library of Congress Cataloging in Publication Data
A catalog record for this book is available from the Library of Congress

Medical knowledge is constantly changing. As new information becomes available, changes in treatment, procedures, equipment and the use of drugs become necessary. The editors and the publishers have, as far as possible, taken care to ensure that the information given in this text is accurate and up to date. However, readers are strongly advised to confirm that the information, especially with regard to drug usage, complies with current legislation and standards of practice.

Commissioning Editor – Laurence Hunter
Project Editor – Michelle Staunton
Project Controller – Frances Affleck
Designer – Sarah Russell
Printed in Spain

The
publisher's
policy is to use
**paper manufactured
from sustainable forests**

Contents

Contents

Contributors

James Aitken MBBS FRCS FCS(SA) FRACS
Senior Lecturer, University of Western Australia, Australia

Dhia Al-Musawi MSc FRCS
Senior Surgical Registrar, Department of Surgery, Chelsea and Westminster
Hospital, London, UK

Stephen George Edward Barker BSc MBBS MS FRCS
Senior Lecturer in Surgery, The Academic Vascular Unit, Department of
Surgery, The Royal Free and University College London Medical School, The
Middlesex Hospital, London, UK

Brian Birch MA MD FRCS
Consultant Urologist, Southampton University Hospitals Trust,
Southampton, UK

Simon Boyes BM FRCS
Vascular Research Fellow, Department of Vascular Surgery, Southampton
General Hospital, Southampton, UK

Jagdeep Chana BSc MD FRCS
Specialist Registrar in Plastic Surgery, Mount Vernon Hospital, Northwood,
Middlesex, UK

Philip Conaghan BA MRCS
Surgical Registrar, Department of General Surgery, Northampton General
Hospital, NN1 5BD, UK

N.E. Dudley MA FRCS FRCS(Ed)
Honorary Consultant Surgeon, The John Radcliffe Hospital, Oxford, UK

Kenneth C.H. Fearon MD FRCS
Professor of Surgical Oncology and Honorary Consultant Surgeon,
Department of Clinical and Surgical Sciences (Surgery), Edinburgh Royal
Infirmary, Edinburgh, UK

D .J. Gouma MD
Professor, Department of Surgery, Academic Medical Center, Amsterdam, The Netherlands

Simon John Hollingsworth BSc PhD MPS
Lecturer in Molecular Medicine, The Academic Vascular Unit, Department of Surgery, The Royal Free and University College London Medical School, The Middlesex Hospital, London, UK

Celia L. Ingham Clark MChir FRCS
Consultant Surgeon, Whittington Hospital, London, UK

C.D. Johnson MChir FRCS
Senior Lecturer and Consultant Surgeon, University Surgical Unit, Southampton General Hospital, Southampton, UK

Marion Jonas FRCS
Research Fellow, Section of Surgery, University Hospital, Queen's Medical Centre, Nottingham, UK

Bryony E. Lovett MChir FRCS
Lecturer, Department of Surgery, University College London, London, UK

Alastair G.W. Moses BSc FRCS
Clinical Research Fellow, Department of Clinical and Surgical Sciences (Surgery), Edinburgh Royal Infirmary, Edinburgh, UK

H. Obertop MD
Head and Professor, Department of Surgery, Academic Medical Center, Amsterdam, The Netherlands

Colm Power MMs FRCSI
Registrar, Department of Surgery, Cork University Hospital, Cork, Ireland

Prakash Ratan FRCS
Associate Specialist, Department of Urology, Southampton University Hospitals Trust, Tremona Road, Southampton SO16 6YD, UK

H. Paul Redmond BSc MCh FRCSI
Chairman, Department of Surgery, Cork University Hospital, Cork, Ireland

Christobel Saunders FRCS
Associate Professor, University Department of Surgery, Royal Perth Hospital, Perth, Western Australia, Australia

John H. Scholefield FRCS ChM
Professor of Surgery, Section of Surgery, University Hospital, Queen's Medical Centre, Nottingham, UK

C.P. Shearman BSc MBBS MS FRCS
Head, Department of Vascular Surgery, Southampton General Hospital, Southampton, UK

Shastri Sookhai BSc MD FRCSI
Senior Registrar, Department of Surgery, Cork University Hospital, Cork, Ireland

Jeff Stamatakis MS FRCS
Consultant Colorectal and General Surgeon, Princess of Wales Hospital, Bridgend, UK

Russell W. Strong CMG FRCS FRACS FACS FRACDS
Professor and Director of Surgery, Princess Alexandra Hospital, Woolloongabba, Queensland, Australia

Jenifer Smith MBBS
Director, South and West Cancer Intelligence Unit, Winchester, UK

I. Taylor MD ChM FRCS
Professor and Head, Department of Surgery, University College London, London, UK

Jeremy N. Thompson MChir FRCS
Consultant Gastrointestinal Surgeon, Department of Surgery, Chelsea and Westminster Hospital, London, UK

Michael Thompson MD FRCS
Department of Surgery, Queen Alexandra Hospital, Portsmouth, UK

Paul Tulley BSc FRCS
RAFT Research Fellow, RAFT Institute of Plastic Surgery, Northwood, Middlesex, UK

Vardhini Vijay MS DNB FRCS
Surgical Registrar, Whittington Hospital, London, UK

David J. Wheatley MD ChM FRCS FRCP
British Heart Foundation Professor of Cardiac Surgery, Royal Infirmary, Glasgow, UK

Dhia Al-Musawi   Jeremy N. Thompson

CHAPTER 1

Intra-abdominal adhesions: formation and management

Adhesions are abnormal deposits of fibrous tissue that occur in the peritoneal, pleural and pericardial cavities. Although some adhesion bands are congenital in origin, most of adhesions are the result of an injury to the lining membrane of these cavities. This chapter examines the magnitude of adhesion-related problems, the pathogenesis of adhesions, their treatment and the current methods of adhesion prevention.

PERITONEAL ADHESION-RELATED DISEASE

In the majority of patients, peritoneal injury occurs as a result of surgery or peritonitis or their combination. In a review of 388 patients with abdominal adhesions, 79% had a history of surgery, 18% had a history of peritoneal infection, and 11% had congenital adhesions.[1] Following laparotomy, 95% of patients have been found to have adhesions at subsequent operations.[2] In most patients, postoperative adhesions do not cause any problem. Some patients, however, develop life-long adhesion-related disease. Intraperitoneal adhesions are a major source of morbidity (Table 1.1), being the commonest cause of small bowel obstruction,[3–5] secondary female infertility and ectopic gestation.[6] They may also cause chronic abdominal and pelvic pain.[7,8]

> **Key point 1**
> • Peritoneal adhesions are common and a cause of major morbidity.

Mr Dhia Al-Musawi MSc FRCS, Senior Surgical Registrar, Department of Surgery, Chelsea and Westminster Hospital, 369 Fulham Road, London SW10 9NH, UK
Mr Jeremy N. Thompson MChir FRCS, Consultant Gastrointestinal Surgeon, Department of Surgery, Chelsea and Westminster Hospital, 369 Fulham Road, London SW10 9NH, UK (for correspondence)

Table 1.1 Abdominal adhesion-related clinical problems

- Small intestinal obstruction
- Secondary female infertility
- Ectopic gestation
- Chronic abdominal and pelvic pain
- Difficult and hazardous re-operations

Small bowel obstruction is the most serious consequence of intra-abdominal adhesions. Retrospective studies have shown that 65–75% of patients who require abdominal re-operation have adhesion-related intestinal obstruction.[9,10] Acute appendicitis and appendectomy are potent causes of adhesions. Analysis of six series[2,4,5,11–13] shows that 680 (36%) of 1897 patients presenting with postoperative adhesional intestinal obstruction had undergone appendectomy. In women, the commonest cause of postoperative intestinal obstruction is a previous hysterectomy.[14,15]

Secondary infertility in women is commonly due to pelvic adhesions. In one retrospective review of laparoscopy performed on 100 consecutive women with chronic pelvic pain, 26% of patients had pelvic adhesions as the only pathological finding and 39% of those with secondary infertility had pelvic adhesions.[7]

EPIDEMIOLOGY AND HEALTHCARE COSTS

There is no evidence that postsurgical adhesion formation is age dependent and, by excluding previous gynaecological procedures, no sex bias in the development of adhesions is observed.[1,16]

Although there have been many individual series of patients with adhesional disease reported, the epidemiology of adhesion-related complications in the general population in Britain remained unclear. However, in 1999, a large retrospective cohort study based on the Scottish National Health Service medical record linkage database was published.[17] All patients who underwent open abdominal or pelvic operation in 1986 were followed for 10 years. Of all re-admissions (21,347), 1209 (5.7%) were directly due to adhesion-related problems and 808 (3.8%) required re-operation. Of all re-admissions, 22.1% occurred in the first year after the initial operation, but re-admissions continued steadily throughout the 10-year period. One in three patients was re-admitted at least twice over the 10-year period, and at least one in 18 re-admissions was directly related to adhesions (for operative or non-operative treatment). This high rate of re-admissions, which steadily increased over a 10 year period, indicates the substantial burden on health resources caused by postoperative adhesion-related disease.

In the same study, the rate of re-admission after initial mid-gut and hind-gut surgery in 1986 was substantially higher than the rates after fore-gut, gynaecological and other abdominal operations (see Table 1.2). This relative adhesion risk following specific operations confirmed the results of other smaller-scale studies.[18] The majority of gynaecological adhesiolysis procedures followed hind-gut surgery rather than fore-gut or upper abdominal operations, probably because of the physical distance between fore-gut operation site and the female reproductive organs.

Table 1.2 Number of hospital readmissions for adhesion-related disorders

Site of initial open surgery	Mid & hind-gut	Fore-gut or other Abdom. operations	Female reprod. tract	Total
No. of patients	12,584	8717	8489	29,790
Rate of re-admissions per 100 initial operations (n)				
Directly related to ahesions	5.1 (643)	3.7 (321)	2.9 (245)	4.0 (1209)
Possibly related to ahesions	28.6 (3596)	24.8 (2165)	29.2 (2479)	27.7 (8240)
Rate of re-admissions complicated by adhesions per 100 initial procedures (n)	36.7 (4622)	52.4 (4567)	31.9 (2709)	39.9 (11,898)
Total rate of readmission (n)	70.4 (8861)	80.9 (7053)	64.0 (5433)	71.6 (21,347)

Data from Ellis et al. [17]

Review of the data from the National Health Service in Scotland, showed the total number of admissions directly related to adhesions in 1994 ($n = 4199$) for Scotland was similar to the total numbers of hip replacements, coronary-artery bypass grafts, appendicectomy or haemorrhoid operations during the same period in the same population,[19] which emphasises the prevalence of adhesion-related disorders.

Key point 2

- Surgery is the commonest cause of peritoneal adhesions.

Adhesions result in a large surgical workload and cost to health care systems.[17,20,21] An epidemiological study in the US showed that 282,000 hospital admissions in 1988 were due to adhesion-related disorders and the cost of in-patient adhesiolysis was $1.18 billion.[21] In 1994, 1% of all US admissions involved adhesiolysis treatment, resulting in $1.33 billion of health care expenditure.[22] A similar report from Sweden confirmed the substantial cost to health care systems.[23]

Key point 3

- Adhesion-related disease poses a large economic burden on the healthcare systems of developed countries.

Table 1.3 Causes of peritoneal injury and adhesion formation

- Operative injury
- Bacterial peritonitis
- Radiotherapy
- Ischaemic injury
- Foreign body reactions, e.g. starch, talc
- Chemical injury

PATHOGENESIS OF ADHESION FORMATION

Intra-abdominal adhesions are usually the result of peritoneal injury. A wide range of recognised inflammatory stimuli can cause peritoneal injury (Table 1.3).[24] In modern clinical practice, iatrogenic operative injury to the peritoneum and/or bacterial peritonitis are the leading causes of intraperitoneal adhesions. Histopathological studies demonstrate a clear sequence of events from injury to the formation of adhesions. Peritoneal inflammation leads to the formation of an inflammatory exudate which contains strands of fibrin. This fibrinous exudate is organised and fibroblast invasion is followed by the deposition of collagen and the formation of permanent fibrous tissue.[25,26] This process is not the inevitable result of peritoneal inflammation because mesothelial surfaces such as the peritoneum possess fibrinolytic activity which, if not impaired, will lyse fibrin within the inflammatory exudate before organisation takes place. This biological sequence is illustrated in Figure 1.1.

PERITONEAL FIBRINOLYSIS

For many years it has been recognised that fibrinous peritoneal adhesions may resolve rather than progress into fibrous adhesions.[27] Experimental and clinical studies have identified the presence of plasminogen-activating activity (PAA) in the mesothelium.[28,29] Biopsies from both visceral and parietal peritoneum taken from different abdominal sites have shown similar levels of

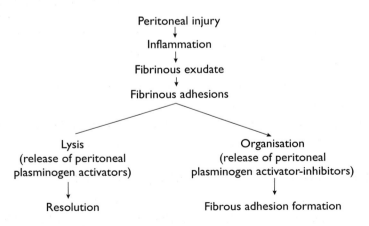

Fig. 1.1 Sequence of adhesion formation.

PAA.[30] Tissue plasminogen activator (tPA) has been found in human peritoneal tissue and is now considered to be the main physiological mediator of PAA.

Effect of peritoneal injury or inflammation on fibrinolytic activity

Animal and human studies have demonstrated that both mechanical and chemical injury reduced peritoneal PAA.[31] This reduction in peritoneal PAA is currently regarded as central to the pathogenesis of adhesion formation. Studies of postoperative peritoneal drain fluid have shown a progressive reduction in PAA in the first few hours following operation, followed by complete loss of fibrinolytic activity up to 72 h after operation.[32]

The reduction in peritoneal PAA caused by injury to peritoneum has been found to be due to the production and release of plasminogen activator inhibitors.[33,34] Both plasminogen activator inhibitors, 1 (PAI-1) and, 2 (PAI-2), have been isolated in high concentration in inflamed peritoneum and also in postoperative peritoneal fluid.[32] These inhibitors reduce and subsequently abolish all peritoneal fibrinolytic activity. It appears that there is a biphasic response to surgery by the peritoneum; an early reduction in peritoneal PAA as a result of loss of t-PA, followed by a later complete loss of fibrinolytic activity as a result of the marked increase in levels of PAI-1 and PAI-2.[32,35]

Using in situ messenger RNA hybridisation techniques, Whawell and co-workers localised PAI-1 production to the mesothelium and the endothelial cells lining the submesothelial blood vessels,[36] and PAI-2 production to the mesothelium and to monocytes within the submesothelial tissue in inflamed peritoneum.[37]

Surgeons have often observed a wide variation among patients in their tendency to form adhesions. Following an equivalent operative procedures, some patients develop extensive, dense and thick adhesions, while others have filmy adhesions limited to the site of surgery. Ivarsson and co-workers have studied this phenomenon and demonstrated, in a prospective clinical study using second-look laparoscopy, that patients who developed severe and dense abdominal adhesions have lower levels of t-PA activity and 10-fold higher PAI-1 levels in their peritoneal fluid compared with those who developed milder and softer adhesions.[38] The same phenomenon was also observed in adhesion tissue taken from patients with varying propensity of adhesion reformation. These observations might explain the individual variation in the susceptibility to adhesion formation. Components of plasmin system within the peritoneum and/or adhesion tissue may be useful predictors for the degree of intraperitoneal adhesion formation or re-formation.

Key point 4

• The peritoneum poses fibrinolytic activity which is lost following injury.

ROLE OF CYTOKINES IN ADHESION FORMATION

During peritoneal inflammation, cytokines and other inflammatory mediators are produced by resident cells (mesothelial, macrophage and fibroblast) and infiltrating leukocytes.[39,40] Inflammatory cytokines have mainly paracrine effects, and their concentrations within the inflamed peritoneal fluid are several 100-fold higher than those in the measured plasma.[39,40]

Studies from mesothelial cells derived from human omentum or from a human mesothelial cell line have demonstrated that the pro-inflammatory cytokines tumour necrosis factor-α (TNF-α), interleukin-1 (IL-1), interleukin-6 (IL-6), and transforming growth factor-β (TGF-β), together with lipopolysaccharide (endotoxin), all resulted in increased PAI-1 release.[41–44]. Studies of postoperative peritoneal fluid following peritoneal injury have shown that the time course of peritoneal cytokine production is in keeping with their de novo stimulation of plasminogen-activator inhibitor production and release.[32] Thus it appears that operative injury results in an increase in peritoneal cytokine production with subsequent stimulation of synthesis and release of plasminogen activator inhibitors. These act to reduce peritoneal fibrinolytic activity and enhance adhesion formation. This concept is supported by two experimental studies, which have shown that postoperative and postirradiation administration of IL-1 increased adhesion formation.[45,46]

Key point 5

- Pro-inflammatory cytokines stimulate peritoneal production of plasminogen activator inhibitors.

MANAGEMENT OF ADHESION-RELATED CLINICAL CONDITIONS

Intraperitoneal adhesions are the commonest cause of small bowel obstruction. Patients with small bowel obstruction are often difficult to assess and require careful evaluation. The management of small bowel obstruction has recently been reviewed.[47] A plain abdominal radiograph frequently provide helpful information on the diagnosis and the possible level of obstruction. Abdominal radiography is normally performed with the patient supine, but erect or lateral images may give additional information in patients with fluid-filled loops of obstructed small bowel. The sensitivity of plain X-ray for the detection of complete intestinal obstruction is reported to be about 50% and may be lower for detection of incomplete intestinal adhesive obstruction.[48] Small bowel enema or follow-through using gastrographin has both a diagnostic and a therapeutic effect, as the hyperosmolar contrast agent stimulates peristalsis and reduces oedema of the bowel wall. In recent years, attention has focused on the potential benefit of computed tomography (CT) enhanced with oral contrast for the diagnosis of adhesive intestinal obstruction. Complete intestinal obstruction caused by adhesions is characterised by air-fluid levels, the absence of mass lesion and a transition zone between dilated prestenotic and empty poststenotic bowel loops. Frager and co-workers compared abdominal radiography and CT in a study of 85 patients.[49] The authors reported a sensitivity of 46% and specificity of 88% for radiography compared to 100% and 83% for CT. In another study, the sensitivity of CT for detection of intestinal ischaemia in strangulated bowel was reported to be 100% (no false negative results) with a specificity of 61%.[50] Magnetic resonance imaging

(MRI) of the gastrointestinal tract has been used for the diagnosis of inflammatory bowel diseases, neoplasms and ischaemia. MRI is usually performed with gadolinium containing oral contrast solutions. The imaging signs of intestinal obstruction on MRI are similar to CT scanning, but the MRI is superior in demonstrating gut wall oedema and peritoneal fluid.

Key point 6

- CT and MR scanning are increasingly helpful in the assessment of patients with small bowel obstruction.

The initial management of adhesive intestinal obstruction is nasogastric suction and correction of fluids and electrolytes. When clinically indicated, the surgical treatment of intestinal adhesion is adhesiolysis. This may be performed either laparoscopically or by laparotomy. There are no prospective randomised trials of laparoscopic versus open surgical adhesiolysis in man to evaluate the incidence of adhesion re-formation at the operated site. Many retrospective studies are limited by inherent selection bias or lack of suitable controls. However, in current practice, laparoscopy is replacing laparotomy as the method of choice for the elective division of pelvic and abdominal adhesions. Laparoscopy is associated with less peritoneal injury, de novo and incisional adhesion formation and has the other advantages of a minimally invasive procedure. Laparoscopic management of adhesive small bowel obstruction is possible in selected cases, for example patients with mild abdominal distension, proximal obstruction or single band obstruction.[51]

Pelvic adhesions are potent causes of secondary female infertility and ectopic pregnancy because of the adhesive occlusion of the fallopian tubes. Peritubal adhesions as a cause of infertility can be detected by hystero-salpingography or visualised at operation. Transvaginal ultrasound scan has recently reported to be useful in the diagnosis of pelvic adhesions.[52]

The relationship between adhesions and chronic pelvic pain is controversial. Using open adhesiolysis, Peters and colleagues showed that women with severe and dense intestinal adhesions had a significant reduction in pain after adhesiolysis compared to those with mild or moderate pelvic adhesions who did not benefit from the procedure.[53] The results of laparoscopic and open (laparotomy) adhesiolysis for women with chronic pelvic pain appear similar, with overall improvement rates of 61% to 89% for laparoscopy and 46% to 71% for laparotomy.[54]

Key point 7 & 8

- Laparoscopic adhesiolysis is widely used, although its role in patients with acute small bowel obstruction remains uncertain.
- The relationship between adhesions and chronic abdominal or pelvic pain is controversial.

PREVENTION OF ADHESION FORMATION

It is important from the prevention point of view, to recognise and define two types of adhesion formation:[55] (i) de novo adhesions that occur where no adhesions existed prior to the operation – either the operative site or at other intraperitoneal locations; and (ii) adhesion re-formation that recur following adhesiolysis – either at the main operative site or at other sites where adhesiolysis has been undertaken.

SURGICAL TECHNIQUE

Good surgical technique remains an important part of adhesion prevention. The principle is to minimise peritoneal injury by careful handling of tissues, the use of atraumatic instruments, starch-free gloves, non-linting swabs, less reactive sutures and, in some procedures, operative magnification. Tissue ischaemia should be avoided and bacterial contamination minimised to avoid postoperative peritoneal infection. Careful haemostasis is an integral part of good surgical technique. Blood clots may adhere to the injured peritoneum and provide the fibrin matrix necessary for adhesion formation.[56] The type of surgical incision is an important factor in adhesion formation. An analysis of 360 women with prior intra-abdominal operations has shown that adhesions are more frequent following midline incision than Pfannenstiel incision and following gynaecological operation than obstetric surgery.[57]

Key point 9

- Adhesions can be prevented by careful surgical technique.

The role of peritoneal fluid irrigation using crystalloid solutions during laparotomy or laparoscopy to reduce adhesion formation is not proven and there is some evidence that these solutions are adhesiogenic.[58] The advantage of carbon dioxide (CO_2) and yttrium-aluminium-garnet (YAG) laser for adhesiolysis and haemostasis to reduce adhesion formation or re-formation remains controversial.[59,60]. The ultrasonic scalpel showed no benefit in reducing adhesions in patients undergoing tubal surgery for infertility.[61]

LAPAROSCOPY VERSUS LAPAROTOMY IN ADHESION FORMATION

There is some evidence from animal and clinical studies that laparoscopic procedures cause fewer abdominal adhesions compared to open operations.[62–65] The possible factors for decreasing adhesions post-laparoscopy are: meticulous technique with the coaxial illumination and magnification, good haemostasis, liberal irrigation, and use of fine electrodes. Gauze swabs, retractors and foreign bodies such as lint and talcum powder are not used in laparoscopic surgery. Prolonged peritoneal exposure to air during laparotomy and subsequent mesothelial desiccation may contribute to de novo adhesion formation at sites remote from the operative procedure. As the peritoneal cavity is normally sterile, warm and wet, peritoneal injury during laparoscopy may be further minimised by using filtered, heated and hydrated insufflating gas instead of the currently used unconditioned dry gas.

A prospective randomised clinical trial reported by Lundorff and colleagues used second-look laparoscopy to evaluate adhesion formation in a 105 women with ectopic pregnancy randomised to either laparoscopy or laparotomy treatment.[66] The authors concluded that laparoscopic surgery induced fewer de novo adhesions and less adhesion formation at the operation site. Recently, Levrant and co-workers have demonstrated that the incidence of incisional adhesions is less with laparoscopic surgery.[67] Some authors have claimed that laparoscopic procedures decrease adhesion reformation, but this conclusion was not supported in a recent careful meta-analysis.[68] Common problems with such studies are the variable timing of second-look laparoscopy and the classification of adhesions severity. Most of the available clinical data comes from gynaecological studies of fallopian tube surgery and there are few data from general surgical laparoscopic procedures.

In summary, laparoscopic procedures appear to reduce incisional and de novo adhesion formation away from the operative site.

Key point 10

- Laparoscopy reduces de novo adhesion formation.

PHARMACOLOGICAL AGENTS TO PREVENT ADHESIONS

A wide variety of pharmacological agents have been used to reduce the peritoneal inflammatory response to injury. Many of these agents were more effective when administered intraperitonealy than systemically. This disparity may be due to limited drug delivery to the sites where adhesions form, which often suffer from ischaemia caused by vascular ligation or cautery. These agents include non-steroidal anti-inflammatory drugs, corticosteroids, histamine antagonists, antioxidants and calcium channel blocking agents. There is experimental data to support the use of many of these drugs although proof of their efficacy in human studies is sparse.[69,70] Prokinetic agents such as cisapride have been used in an attempt to stimulate peristalsis and prevent small bowel adhesions, but with no clear evidence of benefit.

A number of new agents have been evaluated using a mini-osmotic pump and have been found to be effective in reducing experimental pelvic adhesions. These include *trans*-retinoic acids (reduce pro-inflammatory cytokine production), dipyridamole (anti-platelet action), lazaroids (reduce lipid peroxidation and reactive oxygen metabolites) and anti-inflammatory peptide-2.[71] The main problem with most of these experiments has been maintaining a localised effect of the agent within the peritoneal cavity for a sufficient length of time to prevent adhesions.

Attempts to reduce fibrin deposition or stimulate peritoneal fibrinolytic activity have had some success. Anticoagulation with heparin or warfarin is effective, but carries the risk of intraperitoneal bleeding. RecHirudin is a potent thrombin inhibitor and has been shown in two animal models effective to reduce peritoneal adhesions.[71] A number of fibrinolytic enzymes have been used including streptokinase, urokinase, plasmin and t-PA. These enzymes can be incorporated into a slow release gel and there is experimental evidence of a localised reduction in adhesion formation.[31]

Key point 11

- Pharmacological approaches to adhesion formation have not been adopted into clinical practice.

SECOND-LOOK LAPAROSCOPY

Early second-look laparoscopy is used by some surgeons to evaluate and lyse intraperitoneal adhesions following gynaecological surgery. The time for division of early adhesions ranges from 2–6 weeks. During this period, de novo adhesions are soft and gelatinous and can be lysed relatively easily with a laparoscopic blunt dissector. The aim of such a policy is to reduce the formation of symptomatic and permanent fibrotic adhesions. The evidence for this approach comes mainly from gynaecological studies of uterine myomectomy or pelvic adhesiolysis for infertility.[72,73] Further clinical studies and randomised trials are required before considering this approach as a routine adhesion prevention method.

ADHESION PREVENTION PRODUCTS FOR PERITONEAL SURGERY

A number of products have been used clinically during abdominal and pelvic operations to prevent adhesions (Table 1.4). The ideal product would be: active throughout the peritoneum, easy to use during laparoscopy and open procedures, infection-free, non-reactive, resorbable, remain active in the presence of blood, cheap and effective in preventing both adhesion formation and reformation. No such product is currently available.

LIQUIDS AND GELS

Ringer's lactate peritoneal lavage has been used for many years to prevent adhesions but is rapidly absorbed and its effectiveness is doubtful. Hyskon (32% dextran in 10% dextrose solution) is a hyperosmolar solution and works by hydrofloatation. It is easy to use but postoperative ascites is common and serious side effects have been reported (Table 1.4).

Sepracoat, (Genzyme) is a bioresorbable, viscous, tissue protective solution composed of 0.4% (w/w) sodium hyaluronate in phosphate buffered saline. This adhesion prevention product has been used topically, during open and endoscopic abdominal and thoracic operations. The material is rapidly resorbed from the peritoneal cavity and excreted within 5 days. A prospective, randomised, blinded, placebo-controlled multicentre gynaecological study has demonstrated that intraperitoneal coating with Sepracoat at the beginning and

Table 1.4 Adhesion prevention products

Product	Composition	Mode of action	Limitations	Clinical evidence of effectiveness	Laparoscopic use
Ringer's lactate	Lactated Ringer's solution	Fluid barrier	Rapidly absorbed. Probably not effective and ? adhesiogenic	+/−	Yes
Hyskon	32% Dextran 70 in 10% dextrose solution	Hyperosmolar fluid that causes hydroflotation of organs	Coagulopathy, anaphylaxis, ascites	++	Yes
Sepracoat®	0.4% Sodium hyaluronate in phosphate buffered saline	Coating solution used to prevent de novo solution	No longer marketed	+	Yes
Intergel (FeHA gel)	Aqueous solution – 0.5% sodium hyaluronate cross-linked by ferric ions to increase its viscosity	Highly viscous solution protects traumatised tissues from adhesional adherence	No FDA approval	+	Yes
Adept	4% Icodextrin	Liquid barrier persists in peritoneal cavity	Limited clinical data so far	+	Yes
Interceed TC7	Oxidised regenerated cellulose	Gelatinous layer separates peritoneal surfaces	Acidic, procoagulant – complete haemostasis required, degradation induces inflammatory reaction. Site specific	+++	Yes
Expanded PTFE (Preclude Surgical Membrane)	Expanded polytetrafluoroethylene	Mechanical barrier separates peritoneal layers	Permanent foreign body, require suturing. Site specific	++	Difficult
Seprafilm/ Seprafilm II	Hyaluronic acid and caboxymethylcellulose	Film adheres to the peritoneum and gelatinises rapidly	Membrane is difficult to handle, limited use laparoscopically. Site specific	+++	Difficult

during laparotomy procedures reduced the incidence, extent and severity of de novo adhesions.[74] Although introduced in Europe for adhesion prevention, it was not approved in the US and has been withdrawn from the European market.

Intergel (FeHA) gel is an adhesion prevention aqueous solution which is composed of sodium hyaluronate that has been ionically cross-linked by the addition of ferric chloride to increase its viscosity and prolong its absorption time from the peritoneal cavity. The role of Intergel has been recently assessed in an international multicentre randomised clinical study.[58] This study involved application of 300 ml of intraperitoneal Intergel at the end of laparotomy procedure (treatment group) or 300 ml of lactated Ringer's solution (control group). Using second-look laparoscopy 6-12 weeks after the initial surgical procedure, this study has demonstrated that Intergel is safe, easy to use and effective in reducing the incidence, extent and severity of both reformed and de novo adhesions throughout the abdominal cavity, as well as those adhesions at the site of direct surgical trauma. The benefit of this product has been confirmed by another clinical multicentre study by Thornton and colleagues.[75] Intergel is available for clinical use in Europe, but not at present in the US.

Adept (4% icodextrin solution) is a new liquid barrier anti-adhesion solution. It is easy to use during laparotomy and laparoscopy and has potential activity throughout the peritoneal cavity. However, there is so far limited clinical evidence for its effectiveness and it is not approved in the US.

Fibrin glue or fibrin sealant is a two component substance that becomes solid shortly after mixing. Like any hydrogel, it can applied easily during laparoscopy and it has been considered as a possible agent to reduce adhesion formation. However, animal and human studies have shown no consistent anti-adhesive effect. The glue is made from pooled plasma of several donors, so there is risk of disease transmission.

MEMBRANE BARRIERS

There has been particular interest in recent years in the use of absorbable or non-absorbable membranes that are applied topically to separate traumatised peritoneal surfaces and prevent adhesion formation or reformation (Table 1.4). The critical period for the action of these compounds is the first 5–7 days following injury. There are randomised controlled clinical trials demonstrating benefit for some of these products and their use as a routine method of preventing intra-abdominal adhesions is likely to increase.[76–78] Three membranes are now approved for routine clinical use. Unlike adhesion prevention solutions, which reduce localised and de novo adhesion formation, the effect of these barriers is limited to the site of placement.

Interceed T7 (Johnson & Johnson Patient Care, Somerville, NJ, USA) is composed of oxidised regenerated cellulose which is used to separate opposing peritoneal surfaces. The material becomes gelatinous within 8 h of application in the peritoneal cavity. This gelatinous layer acts to protect the damaged peritoneum from adhesion formation. Interceed is slowly absorbed from the peritoneal cavity over 28 days. The efficacy and safety of Interceed has been shown in a prospective randomised clinical trial.[79] The benefit of

Interceed was also supported by multicentre studies in Japan (open procedures) and Germany (laparoscopic procedures).[80,81] Interceed is a procoagulant and can induce fibrin deposition in the presence of blood within the peritoneal cavity, so complete haemostasis is required before its topical application. The material is acidic, and may have a damaging effect on cells and its degradation involves an inflammatory reaction.

Expanded polytetrafluoroethylene (ePTFE; Gore-Tex Surgical Membrane, W.L. Gore & Associates, Flagstaff, AZ, USA) is a synthetic, non-reactive, non-absorbable mechanical barrier which has been utilised extensively as a pericardial, diaphragmatic and peritoneal substitute. The effectiveness of PTFE in the prevention of localised adhesions has been shown in two large prospective multicentre studies reported the Surgical Membrane Study Group and the Myomectomy Adhesion Study Group.[82,83] Haney and co-workers have reported that the reduction of adhesions by PTFE is superior to Interceed in man.[84] The disadvantages of this product are the presence of a permanent foreign body in the peritoneal cavity and the requirement for suture fixation of the membrane which can be difficult at laparoscopy.

Seprafilm (Genzyme Corp, Cambridge, MA, USA) is a bioresorbable membrane composed of hyaluronic acid and carboxymethylcellulose which is non-toxic, non-immunogenic and biocompatible. The product comes in thin sheets that are applied topically over the damaged peritoneal surfaces. The material adheres well to moist surfaces, gelatinises rapidly and remains in situ up to 28 days. Unlike Interceed, Seprafilm is not a procoagulant and is an effective anti-adhesion product even in the presence of blood. There are two randomised, controlled clinical trials, which demonstrate the benefit of Seprafilm in reducing localised intra-abdominal adhesion formation in gynaecological and colorectal surgery.[76,78] However, Seprafilm membrane requires careful application at open operation and is difficult to use laparoscopically.

Key point 12 & 13

- Absorbable and non-absorbable membrane barriers have been proven to reduce adhesion formation.
- Liquid gels and solutions may have a role in non-site specific adhesion prevention.

THE FUTURE OF ADHESION PREVENTION

Many adhesion prevention products are still under development. Some of these are improvements of the previously tested materials. The plasticised and the more flexible Seprafilm II may be useful in laparoscopic adhesion prevention. Many new formulations of hyaluronic acid (HA) are currently under development such as Hylagel, which consists of two spongelike membranes of cross-linked HA fibres and Sepragel, which is a complexed form of HA. Adhesion prevention products based on synthetic absorbable polymers are being currently evaluated, one example is a polylactic acid/polyethylene glycol (PLA/PEG) co-polymer named Resolve, a viscous gel designed for use in gynaecological and general surgery.[85] A new technology is to incorporate photopolymerisable moieties such as polyethylene oxide which allow an adhesion prevention gel to be delivered to the surgical site laparoscopically and then bonded to it by exposure to a light source.[86] Local drug delivery systems are being developed to prevent adhesions in specific anatomical sites.[71]

Another area of current interest is the selective targeting of damaged peritoneal surfaces by adhesion prevention agents. Current adhesion prevention liquids are used in large quantities in order to coat areas of injured peritoneum as well as the intact peritoneal surfaces. Thus, the effect of the fibrinolytic activity of the normal peritoneum is reduced. An agent that selectively targeted the traumatised tissues would be preferable and a novel 'brush copolymer' has been recently studied.[87] This material consists mainly of a positively charged poly-L-lysine (PLL), which adheres to denuded serosal tissue.

Better understanding of the pathophysiology of peritoneal fibrinolytic activity and adhesiogenesis has stimulated an increased interest in the investigation new biological methods of adhesion prevention. There is evidence that adhesion formation can be reduced through either manipulation of macrophage and/or mesothelial cell function or the use of agents that transform growth factors or reduce cytokine synthesis, secretion or activity. Other interventions may be derived from the work on tissue factor pathways, cell adhesion molecules such as intergins and manipulation of hormone receptors in adhesion tissue.

Key point 14

- New methods of adhesion prevention are being developed.

SUMMARY

Adhesions are a major problem for all surgeons. Peritoneal injury, from a variety of causes, leads to peritoneal inflammation and with it the production of plasminogen activator inhibitors. These inhibitors result in the loss of normal mesothelial fibrinolytic activity and, if prolonged, this allows the organisation of fibrinous adhesions into permanent fibrous adhesions. Small bowel obstruction, secondary female infertility, ectopic pregnancy, chronic abdominal and pelvic pain are the major life-long clinical consequences for the patients with intra-abdominal adhesive disease. Management of these adhesion-related clinical problems result in a large surgical workload and cost to health care systems. Appendicitis and appendectomy are the commonest causes of intra-abdominal adhesions. In women, hysterectomy is also a potent cause of subsequent pelvic adhesive disease. Small and large bowel operations have a higher risk of producing clinically significant adhesion formation. There is good evidence that laparoscopic adhesiolysis is safe, and it may be effective in reducing abdominal and pelvic pain in selected patients.

Intra-abdominal adhesions may be prevented by minimising injury and there is increasing evidence that laparoscopic surgery is an important method of adhesion prevention. There is also an increasing acceptance of the role of adhesion prevention products. A wide variety of products has been used experimentally and clinically to prevent adhesion formation following surgery. Many of the current products are based on hyaluronic acid preparations. Interest is currently focused on the use of bioresorbable membranes which allow localised adhesion prevention. Liquids and gels are also being increasingly used and have the advantages of a more wide-spread area of action and increased ease of use, particularly during laparoscopic operations. Significant advances have been made in the science of adhesion prevention and the development of adhesion prevention products. Further advances are likely over the next few years.

Key points for clinical practice

- .Peritoneal adhesions are common and a cause of major morbidity.

- Surgery is the commonest cause of peritoneal adhesions.

- Adhesion-related disease poses a large economic burden on the healthcare systems of industrialised countries.

- The peritoneum poses fibrinolytic activity which is lost following injury.

- Pro-inflammatory cytokines stimulate peritoneal production of plasminogen activator inhibitors.

- CT and MR scanning are increasingly helpful in the assessment of patients with small bowel obstruction.

- Laparoscopic adhesiolysis is widely used, although its role in patients with acute small bowel obstruction remains uncertain.

- The relationship between adhesions and chronic abdominal or pelvic pain is controversial.

- Adhesions can be prevented by careful surgical technique.

- Laparoscopy reduces de novo adhesion formation.

- Pharmacological approaches to adhesion formation have not been adopted into clinical practice.

- Absorbable and non-absorbable membrane barriers have been proven to reduce adhesion formation.

- Liquid gels and solutions may have a role in non-site specific adhesion prevention.

- New methods of adhesion prevention are being developed.

References

1. Perry Jr JF, Smith GA, Yonehiro EG. Intestinal obstruction caused by adhesions. A review of 388 cases. Ann Surg 1955; 142: 810–816.

2. Menzies D, Ellis H. Intestinal obstruction from adhesions: how big is the problem? Ann R Coll Surg Engl 1990; 72: 60–63.
3. Thompson JN, Whawell SA. The pathogenesis and prevention of adhesion formation. Br J Surg 1995; 82: 3–5.
4. McEntee G, Pender D, Mulvin D et al. Current spectrum on intestinal obstruction. Br J Surg 1987; 154: 283–287.
5. Fuzun M, Kaymak E, Harmancioglu O, Astarcioglu K. Principal causes of mechanical bowel obstruction in surgically treated adults in Western Turkey. Br J Surg 1991; 78: 202–203.
6. Herschlag A, Diamond MP, DeCherney AH. Adhesiolysis. Clin Obstet Gynecol 1991; 34: 395–401.
7. Rapkin AJ. Adhesions and pelvic pain: a retrospective study. Obstet Gynecol 1986; 68: 13–15.
8. Bronson RA, Wallach EE, Lysis or periadnexal adhesions for correction of infertility. Fertil Steril 1977; 278: 613–619.
9. Menzies D. Prospective adhesions: their treatment and relevance in clinical practice. Ann R Coll Surg Engl 1993; 75: 147–153.
10. Ellis H. The magnitude of adhesion-related problems. Ann Chir Gynaecol 1998; 87: 9–11.
11. Bevan PG. Adhesive obstruction. Ann R Coll Surg Engl 1984; 66: 164–169.
12. Raf LE. Causes of abdominal adhesions in cases of intestinal obstruction. Acta Chir Scand 1969; 135: 73–76.
13. Tanphiphat C, Chittmittrapap S, Prasopsunti K. Adhesive small bowel obstruction; a review of 321 cases in a Thai hospital. Am J Surg 1987; 154: 283–287.
14. Ratcliff JB, Kapernick P, Brook GG et al. Small bowel obstruction of gynaecologic surgery. South Med J 1983; 76: 1349–1360.
15. Strickler B, Blanco J, Fox HE. The gynecologic contribution to intestinal obstruction in females. J Am Coll Surg 1994; 178: 617–623.
16. Weibel MA, Majno G. Peritoneal adhesions and their relation to abdominal surgery. A postmortem study. Am J Surg 1973; 126: 345–353.
17. Ellis H, Moran BJ, Thompson JN et al. Adhesion-related hospital readmissions after abdominal and pelvic surgery: a retrospective cohort study. Lancet 1999; 353: 1476–1480.
18. Ellis H. The clinical significance of adhesions: focus on intestinal obstruction. Eur J Surg 1997; 163 (Suppl 577); 5–9.
19. National Health Service in Scotland. Information and Statistics Division: Scottish Health Statistics 1996. Edinburgh: Information and Statistics Division, 1996; 38: 50–51.
20. Scott-Coombes DM, Vipond MN, Thompson JN. Surgeons attitudes to the treatment and prevention of abdominal adhesions. Ann R Coll Surg Engl 1993; 75: 123–128.
21. Ray NF, Larsen Jr JW, Stillman RJ et al. Economic impact of hospitalisations for lower abdominal adhesiolysis in the United States in 1988. Surg Gynecol Obstet 1993; 176: 271–276.
22. Ray NF, Denton WG, Thamer M et al. Abdominal adhesiolysis: inpatient care and expenditure in the United States in 1994. J Am Coll Surg 1998; 186: 1–9.
23. Ivarsson ML, Holmdahl L, Franzjet G, Reisberg B. Cost of bowel obstruction resulting from adhesions. Eur J Surg 1997;163: 679–684.
24. Thompson JN. Peritoneal fibrinolysis and adhesion formation. In: diZerega GS. (ed) Peritoneal Surgery. New York: Springer, 2000; 133–142.
25. Johnson FR, Whiting HW. Repair of parietal peritoneum. Br J Surg 1962; 49: 653–660.
26. Raftery AT. Regeneration of parietal and visceral peritoneum: an electron microscopical study. J Anat 1973; 115: 375–392.
27. Benzor Von H, Blümel G, Piza F. Über Zusammenhänge zwischen fibrinolyse und intraperitonealen adhäsionen. Weiner Klin Wochenschr 1963; 75: 881–883.
28. Raftery AT. Method for measuring fibrinolytic activity in a single layer of cells. Br J Surg 1977; 64: 825–826.
29. Merlo M, Fausone G, Barbero C et al. Fibrinolytic activity of human peritoneum. Eur Surg Res 1980; 12: 433–438.
30. Thompson JN, Paterson-Brown S, Harbourne T et al. Reduced human peritoneal plasminogen-activating activity: a possible mechanism of adhesion formation. Br J Surg 1989; 76: 382–384.

31. Vipond MN, Whawell SA, Thompson JN et al. Effect of experimental peritonitis and ischaemia on peritoneal fibrinolytic activity. Eur J Surg 1994; 160: 471–477.

32. Scott-Coombes DN, Whawell SA, Vipond MN et al. The human intraperitoneal fibrinolytic response to elective surgery. Br J Surg 1995; 82: 414–417.

33. Vipond MN, Whawell SA, Thompson JN et al. Peritoneal activity and intra-abdominal adhesions. Lancet 1991; i: 1120–1122.

34. Whawell SA, Vipond MN, Scott-Coombes DM et al. Plasminogen activator inhibitor-2 inhibits peritoneal fibrinolytic activity in inflammation. Br J Surg 1993; 80: 107–109.

35. Holmdahl L, Eriksson E, Eriksson B, Risberg B. Depression of peritoneal fibrinolysis during operation is a local response to trauma. Surgery (St Louis) 1998; 123: 539–544.

36. Whawell SA, Wang Y, Fleming KA et al. Localisation of plasminogen activator inhibitor-1 production in inflamed appendix by in situ mRNA hybridisation. J Pathol 1993; 169: 67–71.

37. Whawell SA, Thompson EM, Fleming KA et al. Plasminogen activator inhibitor-2 expression in inflamed appendix. Histopathology; 1995; 27: 75–78.

38. Ivarsson ML, Bergström M, Eriksson E, Risberg B, Holmdahl L. Tissue markers as predictors of post-surgical adhesions. Br J Surg 1998; 85: 1549–1554.

39. Badia JM, Scott-Coombes DN, Whawell SA et al. Peritoneal and systemic cytokine response to laparotomy. Br J Surg 1996; 83; 347–348.

40. Ivarsson ML, Holmdahl L, Eriksson E, Soderberg R, Reisberg B. Expression and kinetics of fibrinolytic components in plasma and peritoneum during abdominal surgery. Fibrinolysis 1998; 21: 61–67.

41. Whawell SA, Scott-Coombes DM, Vipond MN, Tebbutt SJ, Thompson JN. Tumour necrosis factor mediated release of plasminogen activator inhibitor-1 by human peritoneal mesothelia cells. Br J Surg 1994; 81: 214–216.

42. van Hinsburgh VWM, Bauer KA, Kooistra T et al. Progress of fibrinolysis during tumour necrosis factor infusion in humans. Concomitant increase in tissue-type plasminogen activator, plasminogen activator inhibitor type-1, and fibrin(ogen) degradation products. Blood 1990; 76: 2284–2289.

43. Tietz EL, Handt S, Elbrecht A et al. Decreased fibrinolytic activity of human mesothelial cells in vitro following stimulation with transforming growth factor-β1, interleukin-1β, and tumour necrosis factor-alpha. In: Treutner K-H, Schumpelick V. (eds) Peritoneal Adhesions. Berlin: Springer, 1997; 146–159.

44. Ivarsson ML, Holmdahl L, Falk P et al. Characterisation and fibrinolytic properties of mesothelial cells isolated from peritoneal lavage. Scand J Clin Lab Invest 1998; 58: 195–203.

45. McBride WH, Mason K, Withers HR et al. Effect of interleukin-1, inflammation and surgery on the incidence of adhesion formation after abdominal irradiation in mice. Cancer Res 1988; 49: 169–173.

46. Herschlag A, Herness IGO, Wimberly HC et al. The effect of interleukin-1 on adhesion formation in the rat. Am J Obstet Gynecol 1991; 4: 141–151.

47. Wilson MS, Ellis H, Menzies D, Moran BJ, Parker MC, Thompson JN. A review of the management of small bowel obstruction. Ann R Coll Surg Engl 1999; 81: 320–328.

48. Gulliver DJ, Backert KA. CT of the small bowel. Appl Radiol 1994; 11: 39–44.

49. Frager D, Medwid SW, Baer JW, Mollinelli B, Freidman M. CT of small bowel obstruction. Am J Roentgenol 1994; 162: 37–41.

50. Donckier V, Closet J, Van Gansbecke D et al. contribution of CT to decision making in the management of adhesive small bowel obstruction. Br J Surg 1988; 85: 1071–1074.

51. Adams S, Wilson T, Brown AR. Laparoscopic management of acute small bowel obstruction. Aust N Z J Surg 1993; 63: 39–41.

52. Guerriero S, Ajossa S, Lai MP, Mais V, Paoletti AM, Melis GB. Transvaginal ultrasonography in the diagnosis of pelvic adhesions. Hum Reprod 1997; 12: 2649–2653.

53. Peters AAW, Trimbos-Kemper GCM, Admiral C et al. A randomised clinical trial on the benefit of adhesiolysis in patients with intraperitoneal adhesions and chronic pelvic pain. Br J Obstet Gynaecol 1992; 99: 59–62.

54. Holschneider CH, DeCherney H. Laparoscopic treatment of peritoneal adhesions. In: diZerega GS. (ed) Peritoneal Surgery. New York: Springer, 2000; 367–378.

55. Pouly J-L, Seak-San S. In: diZerega GS. (ed) Peritoneal Surgery. New York: Springer, 2000; 183–192.

intra-abdominal adhesions: formation and management

56. Gomel V. Peritoneal fibrinolysis and adhesion formation. In: diZerega GS. (ed) Peritoneal Surgery. New York: Springer, 2000; vii–xi.

57. Nezhat CR, Nezhat FR, Luciano AA et al. Laparoscopy. In: Nezhat CR, Nezhat FR, Luciano AA, Siegler Am, Metzger DA, Nezhat CH. (eds) Operative Gynaecologic Laparoscopy: Principles and Techniques. New York: McGraw-Hill, 1995; 79–96.

58. Wiseman DM, Trout JR, Diamond MP. The rates of adhesion developments and the effects of crystaloid solutions on adhesion development in pelvic surgery. Fertil Steril 1998; 70: 702–711.

59. Diamond MP, Daniell JF, Martin DC et al. Tubal patency and pelvic adhesions at early second look laparoscopy following intra-abdominal use of the carbon dioxide laser: initial report of intra-abdominal laser study group. Fertil Steril 1984; 42: 717–723.

60. Filmar S, Gomel V, McComb P. The effectiveness of CO_2 laser and electromicrosurgery in adhesiolysis: a comparative study. Fertil Steril 1986; 45: 407–411.

61. Tulandi T, Chan KL, Arseneau J. Histopathological and adhesion formation after incision using ultrasonic vibrating scalpel and regular scalpel in the rat. Fertil Steril 1994; 61: 548–550.

62. Lundorff P, diZerega GS, John DB et al. Clinical evaluation of Intergel adhesion prevention solution for the reduction of adhesion following peritoneal cavity surgery; an international multicentre study of safety and efficacy. Abstract No. 0-069. European Society of Hormones and Reproductive Endocrinology (ESHRE), Goteborg, Sweden, 1998.

63. Bulletti C, Polli V, Negrinin V, Giacomucci E, Flamigni C. Adhesion formation after laparoscopic myomectomy. Am J Assoc Gynecol Laparosc 1996; 3: 533–536.

64. Marana R, Luciano AA, Muzii I. Laparoscopy versus laparotomy for ovarian conservative surgery: a randomised trial in the rabbit model. Am J Obstet Gynecol 1994; 171: 861–864.

65. Filmar F, Gomel V, Macomb P. Operative laparoscopy versus abdominal surgery: a comparative study on post-operative adhesion on the rat model. Fertil Steril 1987; 48: 486–489.

66. Lundorff P, Hahlin M, Kallfelt B, Thorburn J, Lindblom B. Adhesion formation after laparoscopic surgery in tubal pregnancy: a randomised trial versus laparotomy. Fertil Steril 1991; 55: 911–915.

67. Levrant SG, Bieber EJ, Barnes RB. Anterior abdominal wall adhesions after laparotomy or laparoscopy. Am J Assoc Gynecol Laparosc 1997; 4: 353-356.

68. Diamond MP, Daniel JF, Johns DA. Adhesion formation and reformation after operative laparoscopy: assessment at early second-look procedures. Fertil Steril 1991; 55: 500–504.

69. diZerega GS. Contemporary adhesion prevention. Fertil Steril 1994; 61: 219–235.

70. Wiseman D. Polymers for the prevention of surgical adhesions. In: Domb AJ. (ed) Polymeric Site-specific Pharmacotherapy. London: Hohn Wiley & Sons, 1994; 369–421.

71. Rodgers KE, diZerega GS. Developing pharmacologic agents for adhesion prevention. In: diZerega GS. (ed) Peritoneal Surgery. New York: Springer, 2000; 441–457.

72. Ugur M, Turan C, Mungan T et al. Laparoscopy for adhesion formation following myomectomy. Int J Gynaecol Obstet 1996; 53: 145–149.

73. Raiga J, Canis M, Le Boudec G et al. Laparoscopic management of adnexal abscesses: consequences of fertility. Fertil Steril 1996; 66: 712–717.

74. Diamond MP. Reduction of de novo postsurgical adhesions by intraoperative precoating with Sepracoat (HAL-C) solution: a prospective randomised, blinded, placebo-controlled multicentre study. The Sepracoat Adhesion Study Group. Fertil Sertil 1998; 69: 1067–1074.

75. Thornton MH, Johns DB, Campeau JC et al. Clinical evaluation of 0.5% ferric hyaluronate adhesion prevention gel for the reduction of adhesion following peritoneal cavity surgery: open-label pilot study. Hum Reprod 1998; 13: 1480–1485.

76. Diamond MP, Seprafilm Adhesion Study Group. Reduction of adhesion after uterine myomectomy by Seprafilm membrane (HAL-F): a blinded, prospective, randomised multicentre clinical study. Fertil Steril 1996; 66: 904–910.

77. Beck DE. The role of Seprafilm bioresorbable membrane in adhesion prevention. Eur J Surg Suppl 1997; 577: 49–55.

78. Becker JM, Dayton MT, Fazio VW et al. Prevention of postoperative abdominal adhesions by a sodium hyaluronate-based bioresorbable membrane: A prospective randomised, double-blinded multicentre study. J Am Coll Surg 1996; 183: 297–306.

79. Interceed (TC7) Adhesion Barrier Study Group. Prevention of post-surgical adhesions by INTERCEED (TC7), an absorbable adhesion barrier: a prospective, randomised multicentre clinical study. Fertil Steril 1989; 51: 933–938.
80. Sekiba K and the Obstetrics and Gynaecology Adhesion Prevention Committee. Use of Interceed (TC7) absorbable adhesion barrier to reduce postoperative adhesion reformation in infertility and endometriosis surgery. Obstet Gynecol 1992; 79: 518–522.
81. Wallwiener D, Meyer A, Bastert G. Adhesion formation of the parietal and visceral peritoneum: an explanation for the controversy on the use of autologous and alloplastic barriers. Fertil Steril 1998; 69: 132–137.
82. Surgical Membrane Study Group. Prophylaxis of pelvic sidewall adhesion formation with Gore-Tex surgical membrane: a multicentre clinical investigation. Fertil Steril 1992; 57: 921–923.
83. Myomectomy Adhesion Study Group. An expanded polytetrafluoroethylene barrier (Gore-Tex surgical membrane) reduces post-myomectomy adhesion formation. Fertil Steril 1995; 57: 921–923.
84. Haney AF, Hesla J, Hurst BS et al. Expanded polytetrafluoroethylene (Gore-Tex Surgical Membrane) is superior to oxidised regenerated cellulose (Interceed TC7) in preventing adhesions. Fertil Steril 1995; 63: 1021–1026.
85. Diamond MP, Rodgers K, Stern T, Cohn D, Pines E, diZerega G, Resolve TM. A solution approach to reduce postoperative adhesions in the rabbit double uterine horn model. Presented at Annual Regional International Society of Gynaecologic Endoscopy (ISGE) meeting. Amsterdam, 1998.
86. Hill-West JL, Chowdhury SM, Sawhney AS, Pathak CP, Dunn RC, Hubbell JA. Prevention of postoperative adhesions in the rat by in situ photopolymerisation of biological hydrogel barriers. Obstet Gynecol 1994; 83: 56–64.
87. Hubbel JA, Hill-West JL, Drumheller PD, Sanghamitra C, Sawhney A. Multifunctional organic polymers. US Patent 5,462,990, 1995.

intra-abdominal adhesions: formation and management

Shastri Sookhai   Colm Power   H. Paul Redmond

SIRS in general surgery

As much as the field of general surgery has evolved and become better defined in recent years, so too has the most challenging condition we encounter in our practice, namely the sepsis syndrome. The term sepsis syndrome, originally coined by Bone in 1989,[1] was applied to a population of patients at risk from adult respiratory distress syndrome (ARDS). It did much to simplify a disconcerting constellation of symptoms and signs and enabled us to better approach and interpret the host response to surgical insults and disease. A pioneering definition, it has inevitably become archaic as our understanding of the human immunological riposte to injury has increased. Newer categories and more precise definitions addressing the pathophysiology of this disease have arisen from a landmark consensus conference.[2] The systemic inflammatory response syndrome (SIRS), implying two or more defined variables (Table 2.1) arising from a non-specific stimulus, is the cardinal manifestation of an inflammatory reaction mounted by the host which may ultimately be more autodestructive than beneficial. Sepsis is described as SIRS with a documented microbial origin. Both SIRS and sepsis are harbingers of multiple organ dysfunction syndrome (MODS) which is defined as failure to maintain homeostasis without intervention. The relevance of these conditions to general surgery is firmly established as they comprise the leading cause of mortality in the surgical intensive care unit.[3] The disease process is usually characterised by the progression of a persistent hyperdynamic, hypermetabolic state to a gradual functional deterioration of multiple organs, e.g. lungs, liver, kidney. As the crucial rate-limiting step in this continuum, the development of SIRS remains the pivotal clinical incident influencing patient outcome. Below, we discuss the

Mr Shastri Sookhai BSc MD FRCSI, Senior Registrar, Department of Surgery, St Luke's General Hospital, Kilkenny, Ireland (for correspondence)
Mr Colm Power MMs FRCSI, Registrar, Department of Surgery, Cork University Hospital, Cork, Ireland
Prof. H. Paul Redmond BSc MCh FRCSI, Chairman, Department of Surgery, Cork University Hospital, Cork, Ireland

Table 2.1 Abbreviated definitions of the systemic inflammatory response syndrome (SIRS) and allied disorders

---

SIRS
Systemic inflammatory response to a variety of severe clinical insults manifested by 2 or more of the following conditions:

Temperature	> 38∞C or < 36∞C
Heart rate	> 90 beats/min
Respiratory rate	> 20 breaths/min **or** $PaCO_2$ < 32 torr (< 4.3 kPa)
White cell count	> 12,000 cells/mm³ **or**
	< 4,000 cells/mm³ **or**
	> 10% immature (band) cells

Sepsis
The systemic response to infection. The response incorporates the same criteria as SIRS but with a documented microbial origin

Severe sepsis
Sepsis associated with organ dysfunction, hypoperfusion or hypotension. Hypoperfusion and perfusion abnormalities may include lactic acidosis, oliguria or alterations in mental status

Septic shock
Sepsis associated with hypotension, despite adequate fluid resuscitation, along with the presence of perfusion abnormalities as listed for severe sepsis. Patients who are on inotropic or vasopressor agents may not be hypotensive in the presence of perfusion abnormalities

---

pathophysiology of SIRS, its principal mediators and effectors, its current status and how these pertain to general surgery.

PATHOPHYSIOLOGY OF SIRS

SIRS is the massive inflammatory reaction resulting from systemic mediator release by activated cells that ultimately may lead to multiple organ dysfunction; thus, it is an extravagant and often lethal inflammatory backlash. It is characterised by an imbalance in pro- and anti-inflammatory activity with subsequently deleterious effects for the host. Localised inflammation confined to a single focus can normally be tightly controlled with few detrimental consequences, but when this regulation is lost, an exaggerated global response ensues which is manifest clinically as SIRS. It has been proposed that there are three stages to SIRS.[4]

SIRS STAGE 1

In response to an injury or infection, the local environment produces cytokines which promote wound repair and the recruitment of phagocytes directed at pathogenic organisms (viruses, bacteria, fungi and protozoa).

SIRS STAGE 2

Small amounts of cytokines are released into the circulation with the common aim of enhancing local defence. This systemic release may be so small as to often be undetectable, but is primarily protective. It cannot be categorised as pathological or imbalanced. These mediators dampen the initial inflammatory response by down-regulating further cytokine production and counteracting the effects of cytokines already released, thus restoring homeostasis.

SIRS STAGE 3

If homeostasis cannot be restored, a massive systemic reaction begins. At this stage, cytokines and other mediators are predominantly autotoxic and may cause profound local and systemic cellular destruction. The systemic damage results from local loss of capillary integrity at distant sites with subsequent mediator spillage out into end-organs precipitating end-organ destruction.

In many patients SIRS progressing to MODS is ascribed to the summation of several insults rather than one event. Each of these insults may be clinically insignificant, but may prime the host immune system so that the inflammatory response to subsequent events becomes exaggerated. This 'two-hit theory' is an attractive concept and may partly explain how infection may convert a non-lethal operative procedure or trauma into a deadly insult. Regardless of the proximal events, the down-stream sequelae of SIRS progressing to MODS are depressingly consistent.

Uncontrolled systemic vasodilation resulting from the action of specific inflammatory mediators (histamine, prostaglandins, etc.) causes a significant, persistent lowering of peripheral vascular resistance and hypotension. The increased vascular permeability induced by similar and more diverse mediators gives rise to profound extravascular third spacing. This often co-exists with depressed myocardial contractility as a consequence of leukocyte-mediated and ischaemic myocyte injury. The preterminal event thus is severe haemodynamic instability, usually refractory to volume and inotropic support, associated with recondite lactic acidosis indicative of impaired perfusion and altered cellular metabolic function. Standard critical care supportive measures, more often than not, are ineffective when confronted with such overwhelming systemic dysfunction.

MEDIATORS OF SIRS

ENDOGENOUS MEDIATORS OF SIRS

Cytokines
These are the physiological messengers of the inflammatory response and the principal molecules involved are tumour necrosis factor α (TNF-α), inter-leukins (IL) IL-1β and IL-6. Cytokines bind to specific receptors on cell surfaces (or in serum) and induce dimerization or polymerization of receptor polypeptides activating intracellular signalling pathways (e.g. kinase cascades) which results in the production of transcription factors. These migrate to the nucleus and bind to enhancer regions of genes induced by that cytokine. For comparative purposes, in SIRS, TNF-α appears to be the first cytokine released systemically (peak at 2 h) followed by IL-1β and IL-6 (peak at 4 h).[5]

Tumour necrosis factor α: This cytokine is thought to be the most important proximal mediator of the inflammatory response. TNF-α appears to be responsible for most metabolic and nutritional changes that occur in catabolic states accounting for its alternative name, cachectin.[6] It is produced primarily by macrophages but also by lymphocytes, natural killer cells and Kupffer cells. The half-life of circulating TNF is 14–18 min in humans. In healthy subjects, plasma levels rarely exceed 35 pg/ml,[7] and at slightly higher concentrations it plays a role in cell proliferation and differentiation and also the regulation of cytokine interaction.[8,9] At these levels, TNF, therefore, induces mechanisms for tissue remodelling, inflammation and cytotoxicity. However, these biological effects of TNF are elicited when only 5–10% of TNF receptors on cells are occupied and it is for this reason when TNF exists in overwhelming amounts, as occurs in SIRS, that we observe tissue injury, irreversible shock and death. The systemic and tissue-specific cellular mechanisms of TNF are dependent on its direct effects as well as the release of other soluble mediators from host cells. It induces IL-1β release from endothelial cells and macrophages, while IL-1β subsequently stimulates the biosynthesis of other cytokines. The presence of IL-1β and these other cytokines appear to enhance the sensitivity of tissues to TNF thereby establishing a vicious circle promulgating the deleterious effects associated with TNF[10] which is characteristic of SIRS. The predominant role of TNF amongst pro-inflammatory cytokines is illustrated in a number of studies which have demonstrated that, in certain surgical scenarios, the concentration of TNF in the bloodstream may be a predictor of survival during invasive infection.[11] It has also been shown that the administration of TNF in healthy subjects results in the physiological and metabolic abnormalities associated with sepsis and SIRS.[7] We have already mentioned that it is the initial cytokine to be released in SIRS suggesting a pre-eminent position for TNF in the hierarchy of endogenous inflammatory mediators. Most significant, however, are the findings demonstrating that blockade of TNF activity with monoclonal antibodies prevents death after lethal Gram-negative bacteraemia in a murine model and TNF deficient or TNF 'knockout' mice are similarly resistant to endotoxic shock.[12]

Interleukin 1β: TNF displays a symbiotic relationship with IL-1, neither existing without a proportionate systemic presence of the other.[13] IL-1 attends in two forms, IL-1α and IL-1β, produced by macrophages, monocytes and to lesser degrees by other cell types. Both are recognised equally by one IL-1 receptor but IL-1β is the predominant form in vivo. In healthy humans, levels of IL-1β remain below 60 pg/ml with a half-life of 6–10 min. Intravenous murine administration of 10–100 ng/ml results in fever, neutrophilia and increased acute-phase protein synthesis.[14] Higher levels induce hypotension, leukopenia, tissue injury and death, i.e. a SIRS-like state. These effects are not as profound as those seen with TNF administration, but IL-1 accounts for significant neutrophil margination, leukocyte binding and procoagulant activity.[15] The pro-inflammatory effects of TNF and IL-1 are cumulative and each stimulates the production of the other indicating that they probably account for the majority of the systemic effects typical of SIRS. As is the case for TNF, animal studies employing blockade of IL-1 activity with receptor antagonists have demonstrated improved survival in Gram-negative bacterial sepsis.[16]

Table 2.2 The principal human cytokines involved in inflammation (excluding TNF, GM-CSF, etc.) are primarily of the interleukin nomenclature as outlined above

Cytokine	Source	Target	Principal effects
IL-1α	Macrophage	Lymphocyte	Phagocyte activation
	Fibroblast	Endothelium	Activates adhesion molecules
	Lymphocyte	Macrophage	Prostaglandin synthesis
			Lymphocyte stimulation
IL-1β	Epithelial cells	Other	Similar effects
	Astrocytes		
IL-2	T cells	T and B cells	T /B cell growth/activation
		NK cells	NK cell activation
IL-3	T cells	Stem cells	Haemopoietic properties
	Thymic cells		
IL-4	Th2 cells	B cells	Activation/division
IL-5	Th2 cells	B cells	Development/differentiation
		Eosinophils	
IL-6	Macrophages	T cells	Growth
	Endothelium	B cells	Differentiation
		Hepatocytes	Acute phase protein synthesis
IL-8	Monocytes	Neutrophils	Activation/chemotaxis
	Endothelium	Monocytes	
IL-9	CD4 T cells	T cells	Division
		Mast cells	Development
IL-10	Th2 cells	Monocytes	Inhibits cytokine synthesis
IL-12	Macrophages	NK cells	Activation
IL-14	T cells	B cells	Proliferation
IL-15	Monocytes	T/B cells	Division
IL-16	CD8+ T cells	CD4+ T cells	Chemotaxis

Interleukin 6: Levels of this cytokine are recognised as being representative of the degree of host inflammatory activity. IL-6 itself belongs to a family of phosphoglycoproteins and is the primary mediator of the altered hepatic acute-phase protein synthesis occurring in SIRS. It is the final common mediator in a cascade of cytokine activity elicited by lipopolysaccharide, TNF and IL-1. Other activities include B cell stimulation, cytotoxic T cell differentiation and PMN accumulation/activation.[17] IL-6 administration does not result in the effects observed with TNF or IL-1; however, when TNF or IL-1 activity is attenuated, the subsequent IL-6 response is suppressed. It has additionally been shown that blockade with anti-IL-6 monoclonal antibodies protects mice from the lethal SIRS state elicited by both *Escherichia coli* and TNF.[18]

Table 2.2 lists the principal human interleukins and their main pro- or anti-inflammatory properties.

Secondary endogenous mediators of inflammation

Prostaglandins and leukotrienes: Derivatives of arachidonic acid, of cyclo- or lipo-oxygenase origin, are potent mediators of SIRS despite significant anti-inflammatory activity. Apart from vasodilatory effects, incurring low systemic vascular resistance and hypotension, they are responsible for a variety of motile cellular events. Produced by endothelial cells, macrophages and neutrophils, PGE_2 is capable of modulating TNF and IL-1 release from a number of cell types whilst concurrently inhibiting T and B cell mitogenesis. TXA_2 induces platelet aggregation and neutrophil accumulation. LTB_4 promotes neutrophil chemotaxis and adhesion to endothelium. Raised levels of PGI_2 correlate with the severity of septic shock illustrating the pertinence of these metabolites to the development and maintenance of SIRS.

Nitric oxide: Arising from the conversion of L-arginine to citrulline by constitutive nitric oxide synthetase (cNOS) or inducible NOS (iNOS) this potent molecule is directly linked with the degree of hypotension seen in SIRS.[19] It influences the inflammatory response by enhancing vasodilation, oedema formation and negative myocardial inotropy contributing significantly to cellular and systemic morbidity. The autotoxic effects result from an iron-dependent dysregulation of cellular respiration and DNA synthesis. Furthermore, endothelial cells are capable of converting nitric oxide to peroxynitrite which is markedly cytotoxic, thus compounding SIRS in certain circumstances.

Reactive oxygen species (ROS): Reactive oxygen species (H_2O_2, HOCl, etc.) are involved in most types of inflammatory tissue injury and are derived primarily from phagocytic leukocytes. Oxidative degradation and altering protease/anti-protease balance are the mechanisms by which superoxide radicals contribute to the cellular destruction accompanying SIRS.

Platelet activating factor (PAF): PAF, derived from a multitude of cells under inflammatory conditions, directly activates cells and increases cellular adhesion. By increasing vasodilation, it lowers arterial blood pressure and is also negatively inotropic. Specific PAF receptor antagonists have been shown to protect dogs from fatal endotoxic shock.[20]

EXOGENOUS MEDIATORS OF SIRS

Lipopolysaccharide (LPS/endotoxin)

This bacterial wall product has long been considered the principal exogenous mediator of inflammation and is a pivotal mediator of the SIRS encountered in the field of general surgery. Structurally, it consists of a highly conserved active lipid A moiety, a variable core oligosaccharide region and an O side chain which collectively exist in the outer membrane of Gram-negative bacteria. It interacts with a variety of cell types via the receptors CD14, CD11/18 and Toll-like receptors 2 and 4. Utilising CD14 to stimulate cells requires the presence of lipopolysaccharide binding protein (LBP) in serum. This enhances cellular responses to LPS and is an innate protective device designed to activate the immune system even in the presence of minute quantities of endotoxin. CD14 also exists in serum and participates in all phases of LPS-induced SIRS due to its ability to induce LPS sensitivity in cells lacking CD14 receptors (e.g. endothelial cells). LPS induces profound TNF and IL-1 release from macrophages via activation of p38, a 38 kDa member of the mitogen activated protein (MAP) kinase family.[21] It has emerged that a number of Gram-negative and Gram-positive bacterial products can initiate a SIRS-like state in animal models and have LPS-like effects in in vitro experiments suggesting that LPS is just one of many molecules which mediate bacterial sepsis.

The gut hypothesis of SIRS has been used to explain why no identifiable focus of infection can be found in as many as 30% of bacteraemic patients who die from SIRS/MODS. Clinical evidence abounds demonstrating that intestinal permeability is increased in patients with SIRS. This facilitates translocation of bacteria colonising the intestinal tract into the mesenteric lymphatics from where they gain systemic access and mediate end-organ damage.

CELLULAR EFFECTORS OF SIRS

NEUTROPHILS (PMN)

These phagocytic leukocytes account for 95% of circulating granulocytes and are the first cells to respond to tissue injury, thus playing a pivotal role in the development of SIRS. PMNs contain powerful oxidative (cytotoxic ROS and reactive nitrogen species) and non-oxidative (degradative granule enzymes, chemotactic proteins and toxic cationic proteins) pathways which are critical to effective killing of invasive pathogens. The PMN is considered the primary cell type responsible for the auto-destructive end-organ damage associated with SIRS. This is because activated PMNs demonstrate delayed apoptosis (programmed cell death) allowing PMNs and their cytotoxic products to persist at sites of inflammation thereby perpetuating tissue injury.

MONOCYTES/MACROPHAGES

These are known as 'professional' phagocytes which remove particulate antigens from inflammatory foci in addition to presenting antigen to T cells. Myeloid progenitors in bone marrow differentiate from promonocytes to blood monocytes, cells from this circulating pool then migrate through blood vessel walls into various organs to become tissue macrophages. They possess intracytoplasmic lysosomes containing peroxidase and acid hydrolases essential for intracellular destruction of micro-organisms. In their activated form, they represent a vast reservoir of the pro-inflammatory cytokines TNF, IL-1 and IL-6 and are major effectors of SIRS.

ENDOTHELIAL CELLS

Owing to their location, these cells have important structural and functional roles both in maintaining homeostasis and regulating the response to injury. They respond to adverse environmental stimuli through the release of large quantities of oxygen free radicals, cytokines and adhesion molecules. Unlike PMNs, endothelial cells, when exposed to LPS and other inflammatory mediators, undergo apoptosis which teleologically is an attractive concept as this prevents the spillage of the cytotoxic compounds which occurs during necrotic cell death. In SIRS, however, the prolonged inflammatory response and failure of PMNs to apoptose results in increased endothelial cell necrosis with concomitant increased vascular permeability and capillary leak syndrome.

Table 2.3 A brief representation of the principal mobile cell types responsible for cell-mediated inflammation

---

Mononuclear phagocyte system

Monocytes/macrophages
See text

Kupffer cells
These are potent phagocytes lining the liver sinusoids. Much of the antigen entering through the gut is removed by these cells

Granulocytes

Neutrophils
See text

Eosinophils
Comprising 2–5% of blood leukocytes, their granules are released by exocytosis and kill pathogens as well as containing anti-inflammatory compounds such as histiminase and aryl sulphatase

Basophils
These constitute < 0.5% of blood leukocytes and possess granules containing inflammatory mediators

Mast cells
Are present in most tissues adjoining the blood vessels. Their granules contain histamine, PAF, prostaglandins and leukotrienes

Lymphoid tissue cells

T cells
In the absence of T cells the host cannot mount cell mediated immune responses. There are two main subsets of T cells: (i) helper T cells (CD4); and (ii) suppressor/cytotoxic T cells (CD8). They collectively recognise foreign antigens, secrete lymphokines and destroy pathogen-infected cells as well as augmenting the B cell-mediated humoral response

B cells
These cells are responsible for antibody production (humoral immunity). On exposure to antigens some B cells differentiate into plasma cells specially adapted for the manufacture/secretion of immunoglobulins

Natural killer cells
Capable of killing a variety of virally infected and transformed target cells to which they have not been previously sensitised.

A variety of other important cell types play major roles in the pathogenesis of SIRS and these are outlined briefly in Table 2.3.

SIRS ARISING FROM CONDITIONS ENCOUNTERED IN GENERAL SURGERY

TRAUMA/HAEMORRHAGE

It has been shown that increased circulating TNF concentrations occur 4 h after trauma and maximal haemorrhage. When haemorrhage is unaccompanied by trauma, the peak is seen 2 h after maximal blood loss. The level of increase is markedly greater when both trauma and haemorrhage co-exist.[22] Conversely, IL-1 levels are undetectable within the first few hours after trauma, which may contribute to the anergy that often occurs in trauma patients. This unexpected phenomenon may be partly explained by the fact that, although overwhelming monocytosis occurs after trauma/haemorrhage, this cell population is characterised by fundamental functional disorders.[23] IL-6 release increases significantly after either trauma or haemorrhage and the cumulative effect incurs an even greater response. This increase occurs within 2 h of injury, may persist for up to 1–3 days and correlates with the volume of blood lost.[24]

PANCREATITIS

TNF appears to be amongst the chief mediators of SIRS in pancreatitis. TNF levels increase markedly and correlate with the degree of pancreatic and pulmonary oedema seen in cerulein-induced pancreatitis.[25] Administration of TNF can induce oedematous enlargement of the pancreas and histology is characterised by PMN and lymphocyte infiltration. In lethal pancreatitis, the terminal stage is heralded by steadily decreasing levels of TNF. IL-6 increases early in the course of pancreatitis and correlates with disease severity to such a degree that it can be used prognostically and to differentiate between severe and mild pancreatitis.[26] IL-1 has been poorly studied in relation to pancreatitis.

PERITONITIS

Septic shock secondary to generalised peritonitis is characterised by systemic release of TNF and IL-6 which is maximal on day one. IL-6 levels remain higher in non-survivors over the first 3 days, whereas IL-1 levels remain unchanged. Patients with documented bacteraemia demonstrate the highest plasma TNF concentrations. There appears to be no difference in cytokine levels and hospital mortality when mono- is compared to polymicrobial peritonitis or acute versus postoperative peritonitis.[27]

OPERATIVE SURGICAL INSULTS

It has been shown that even relatively minor surgical insults, such as skin incision and catheterisation, are sufficient to induce IL-6 release.[28] This finding holds true even when these procedures are performed in an aseptic fashion. IL-6 levels peak at the point of maximal haemorrhage after laparotomy with TNF concentrations doing so 4 h later.[22] The frequency rate and duration of SIRS after surgery is related to the duration and complexity of the operative procedure. These parameters are greater after oesophagectomy, hepatectomy and pancreatoduodenectomy as compared to colorectal resection and cholecystectomy. As one would expect, SIRS criteria decrease over the normal postoperative convalescent period. The appearance of SIRS after postoperative day 3 is suggestive of significant postoperative morbidity such as intracavitary abscess, with one group reporting a 98% specificity with regard to this in their study.[29] We have demonstrated that general anaesthesia and surgery combined causes a significant delay in PMN apoptosis, a major contributor to the development of SIRS, and that it is circulating granulocyte macrophage colony-stimulating factor (GMC-SF) which accounts for this delay in patients with SIRS.[30]

CURRENT STATUS

Despite extensive investigation, clearer understanding and the application of myriad immunomodulatory strategies, the unabated progression from SIRS to MODS continues to herald the demise of a significant sub-population of surgical patients. The most effective measures we can employ remain directed at preventing the development of SIRS or attenuating the advancement to MODS. This treatment is time-honoured and addresses three crucial phases of the care of patients with surgical disease.

RESUSCITATION

Aggressive volume resuscitation is mandatory in the early stages of treatment. Because haemorrhagic or septic shock represents a global ischaemia or reperfusion insult, the primary goal of resuscitation of critically ill patients is to restore and maintain optimal tissue perfusion and oxygenation. Airway protection, adequate ventilation and restoration of normal circulation are the mainstays of immediate resuscitation. Subsequently, appropriate monitoring of volume introduced and being lost, base deficit measurements and correction, use of pulmonary artery catheters and calculation of oxygen delivery and consumption etc. must be commenced.

OPERATIVE INTERVENTION

Whether surgery is required as emergency intervention (e.g. aneurysm repair, abdominal trauma, perforated viscus) in established SIRS or semi-electively for diagnosis and/or prevention of SIRS/MODS, the same basic principles apply in order to minimise adverse immunological sequelae. In selected abdominal trauma situations, early and aggressive treatment of specific injuries may prevent or limit the excess immune response of the host to injury and the re-establishment of homeostasis can be hastened. Infection and excessive activation of the inflammatory system predisposes to SIRS; therefore, removal of all dead or infected tissue in addition to decreasing the likelihood of postoperative infection lowers the bacterial burden in surgical and traumatic wounds. In some instances, damage-control surgery with expeditious repair of vascular injuries, gastrointestinal interruption, abdominal packing and rapid closure allows rapid transfer to intensive care thereby allowing the cardinal elements of resuscitation to be resumed. It has been shown that prudent, early cessation of operative intervention reduces the risk of SIRS/MODS and improves patient outcome.[31] It is also essential that extreme vigilance be exercised in the early treatment of trauma patients thereby preventing the risk of a missed injury, a tenet which persists to meticulous intra-abdominal examination at laparotomy. The very nature of surgery demands that particular attention be paid to patients in the postoperative phase which allows the early identification of secondary complications necessitating early re-operative surgery. The persistent presence of occult tissue necrosis and infection after initial trauma or laparotomy for sepsis continually stimulates the immune response, increasing the risk for SIRS and MODS.

INTENSIVE CARE

It is vital that surgeons maintain alertness after their patients have been transferred to ICU. As the individuals with first-hand experience of the precise nature of the primary insult, consequences and operative treatment we are integral care providers in the postoperative period. Additionally, because infection contributes to the development of SIRS/MODS in at least 50% of patients, all wounds and incisions should be frequently examined for evidence of necrosis and suppuration. Constant attention to nutritional support, antibiotic use, specific organ support and general postoperative resuscitation are necessarily within the province of general surgeons who should work in close alliance with intensivists at all times.

IMMUNOMODULATORY STRATEGIES

As our understanding of the inflammatory reaction to a variety of systemic insults deepens, it has become apparent that modulation of specific pathways or manipulation of certain responses may provide tangible methods of attenuating SIRS. Much energy and industry has been invested in developing these potential therapeutic options. What has become abundantly clear from the results of numerous clinical trials assessing the efficacy of a variety of immunomodulators is that the use of specific agents targeting individual mediators does not adequately address the multifactorial nature of SIRS.

In preceding sections, we have identified the crucial roles played by a number of inflammatory mediators by illustrating how their blockade promotes survival in specific animal or in vitro models of SIRS. Below we provide a short appraisal of how these agents have performed when applied to clinical, human scenarios.

ANTI-TUMOUR NECROSIS FACTOR AGENTS

Despite encouraging results from animal studies, there are contradictory data pertaining to human trials. Antibodies directed at TNF have decreased the 3-day mortality rate in humans, although there was no decrease in the rate of mortality at 28 days between treated and non-treated groups.[32] A phase II and one phase III trial of anti-TNF monoclonal antibody demonstrated no difference in survival between test and control groups. Of note in the phase II trial, it transpired that patients administered medium-to-high doses of the antibody had less favourable outcomes than the placebo group.[33]

ANTI-INTERLEUKIN 1 AGENTS

Human recombinant IL-1ra (receptor antagonist) has been investigated in a randomised phase II trial in 99 patients with sepsis. Mortality at 28 days improved with treatment only if patients with a > 24% risk of death were treated within 2 days of the onset of SIRS. There was no benefit if the patient had a risk of death below 24%. A subsequent trial with a greater number of patients exhibiting sepsis and septic shock failed to support these results.[34]

ANTI-LIPOPOLYSACCHARIDE AGENTS

Antibiotics certainly have a reductive impact on morbidity and mortality related to surgical infection, but in established SIRS their role is limited as systemic cellular activation has already occurred and even dead or non-replicating bacteria are capable of profound antigenic activity. De-activating the pertinent moiety of lipopolysaccharide (lipid A) or lesser moieties, though logical, has similarly led to disappointment. Two of the most eagerly anticipated trials of anti-endotoxin monoclonal antibodies (HA-1A and E-5) appeared to demonstrate benefits, but in depth analysis revealed that only spurious sub-sets of patients had questionable survival advantages conferred. Taurolidine, a non-specific LPS antagonist has no beneficial therapeutic effect on the outcome of sepsis in humans as measured by resolution of organ failure and 28-day mortality rate.[35] It has transpired that many bacterial products can elicit an inflammatory response, thus targeting one above many others present in the bacterial wall is an inherently flawed approach which may account for the limited success observed.

MISCELLANEOUS AGENTS

Cytokine synthesis can be blocked at a translational level by steroids which address TNF-mRNA translation in macrophages, but must be administered pre-emptively. Pentoxifyline, a phosphodiesterase inhibitor, interrupts intracellular signalling and in humans at a pre-translational level decreases TNF and PMN activity during septic shock without affecting overall outcome. Arachidonic acid metabolites mediate haemodynamic alterations in SIRS but COX antagonists, such as indomethacin and ibuprofen, have no effect in modulating outcome in man. Similarly, the use of anti-PAF strategies have been shown to be ineffective in patients.

MINIMALLY INVASIVE SURGERY

The advent of laparoscopy has impacted hugely on general surgical practice from a number of perspectives. The most striking benefits have been reduced postoperative pain, shorter hospital stay and better cosmesis at the cost of increased technical demands and greater expense. It has recently become apparent that laparoscopy yields a lower incidence of surgical infection and SIRS than open surgery. Differential factors that may modify bacterial and human biology and explain these findings include CO_2 pneumoperitoneum, less dessication of intra-abdominal structures, fewer temperature changes, fewer changes in endocrine metabolic function and improved pulmonary function. These variables contribute to a better preserved peritoneal and systemic immune response promoting resolution of inflammation, lesser incidence of SIRS and more rapid recovery.[36,37]

NEW CONCEPTS

SIRS, as already said, represents a disparate collective which surgeons encounter all too frequently in practice. Our overall understanding of this phenomenon remains limited and newer terminologies referring to more refined and specific aspects of the systemic response testify to these limitations. SIRS we fully appreciate is pro-inflammatory in nature but the immune response is often not as discriminate as we would like, hence other definitions have arisen describing a compensatory anti-inflammatory response (CARS), a mixed antagonist response syndrome (MARS) and CHAOS (cardiovascular shock, homeostasis, apoptosis, organ dysfunction and immune suppression). These occupy relevant places in the natural history of SIRS, but are beyond the scope of this remit.

CONCLUSIONS

The ever-increasing incidence of sepsis/SIRS, progressive development of antibiotic resistance among common bacterial pathogens and the limited therapeutic options available provide the stimulus for the continued efforts to develop anti-sepsis agents. The intrinsic complexities of human sepsis/SIRS make it inevitable that effective strategies will necessitate a multi-component approach combining methodologies which address the host cell–pathogen interactions as much as improving physiological support and operative technique. The immunology of SIRS is an exciting field and the global picture is still incompletely understood. Attempts at modulating SIRS, therefore, remain in their infancy; however, with the necessary application and industry, continued research in this area will undoubtedly yield knowledge and information which will ultimately revolutionise the treatment of SIRS of surgical, and more diverse origins.

Key points for clinical practice

- SIRS and sepsis are harbingers of multiple organ dysfunction syndrome (MODS)

- SIRS/MOD are major causes of mortality in the surgical ICU

- TNF-α, IL-1β and IL-6 are principal endogenous mediators of SIRS

- LPSs are major exogenous mediators of SIRS

- Neutrophils, monocytes, macrophages, and endothelial cells are the main cellular effectors of SIRS

- SIRS arises from certain general surgical insults such as: trauma/haemorrhage, pancreatitis, peritonitis and operative surgical insult

- Novel immunomodulatory stategies may prove to be beneficial in attenuating SIRS.

References

1. Bone R C, Fisher Jr C J, Clemmer T P, Slotman G J, Metz C A, Balk R A. Sepsis syndrome: a valid clinical entity. Crit Care Med 1989; 17: 389–393.
2. American College of Chest Physicians-Society of Critical Care Medicine Consensus Conference. Definitions for sepsis and organ failure and guidelines for the use of innovative therapies in sepsis. Crit Care Med 1992; 20: 864–875.
3. Maship L, McMillen R, Brown J. The influence of sepsis and multi-system organ failure on mortality in the surgical intensive care unit. Ann Surg 1984; 50: 94–101.
4. Bone R C. Toward a theory regarding the pathogenesis of the systemic inflammatory response syndrome: what we do and do not know about cytokine regulation. Crit Care Med 1996; 24: 163–171.
5. Dofferhoff A S M, Bom V J J, de Vries-Hospers H G et al. Patterns of cytokines, plasma endotoxin, plasminogen activator inhibitor, and acute-phase proteins during the treatment of severe sepsis in humans. Crit Care Med 1992; 20: 185–192.
6. Kawakami M, Pekala P H, Lane M D et al. Lipoprotein lipase suppression in 3T3-L1 cells by an endotoxin-induced mediator from exudate cells. Proc Natl Acad Sci USA 1982; 79: 912–916.
7. Michie H R, Manogue K R, Spriggs D R et al. Detection of circulating tumour necrosis factor after endotoxin administration. N Engl J Med 1988; 318: 1481–1486.
8. Ming W J, Bersani L, Mantovani A. Tumour necrosis factor is chemotactic for monocytes and polymorphonuclear leukocytes. J Immunol 1987; 138: 1468–1474.
9. Sugarman B J, Aggarwal B B, Hass P E et al. Recombinant human tumour necrosis factor-a: effects on proliferation of normal and transformed cells in vitro. Science 1985; 230: 943–946.
10. Okusawa S, Gelfrand J A, Ikejima T, Connolly R J, Dinarello C A. Interleukin-1 induces a shock-like state in rabbit. Synergism with tumour necrosis factor and the effect of cyclooxygenase inhibition. J Clin Invest 1988; 81: 1162–1172.
11. Damas P, Ledoux D, Nys M et al. Cytokine serum levels during severe sepsis in humans: IL-6 as a marker of severity. Ann Surg 1992; 215: 356–362.
12. Roitt I, Brostoff J, Male D. In: Immunology, 5th edn. Somerset, UK: Mosby International, 1998; 121–138.
13. Dinarello C A. Interleukin-1. Rev Infect Dis 1984; 6: 51–95.
14. Dinarello C A. Interleukin-1 and interleukin-1 antagonism. Blood 1991; 8: 1627–1652.
15. Nawroth P P, Handley D A, Esmon C T, Stern D M. Interleukin-1 induces endothelial cell procoagulant while suppressing cell-surface anticoagulant activity. Proc Natl Acad Sci USA 1986; 83: 2460–2464.
16. Pruitt J H, Copeland E M I, Moldawer L L. Interleukin-1 and interleukin-1 antagonism in sepsis, systemic inflammatory response syndrome and septic shock. Shock 1995; 3: 235–251.
17. Davies M G, Hagen P O. Systemic inflammatory response syndrome. Br J Surg 1997; 84: 920–935.
18. Starnes Jr H F, Pearce M K, Tewari A, Yim J H, Zon J C, Abrams J S. Anti-IL-6 monoclonal antibodies protect against lethal Escherichia coli infection and lethal tumour necrosis factor-α challenge in mice. J Immunol 1990; 145: 4185–4191.
19. Brady A J, Poole-Wilson P A. Circulatory failure in septic shock. Nitric oxide: too much of a good thing? Br Heart J 1993; 70: 103–105.
20. Moore J M, Earnest M A, DiSimone A G, Abumrad N N, Fletcher J R. A PAF antagonist BN 52021, attenuates thromboxane release and improves survival in lethal canine endotoxaemia. Circ Shock 1991; 35: 53–59.
21. Han J, Lee J D, Bibbs R, Ulevitch R J. A MAP kinase targeted by endotoxin and hyperosmolarity in mammalian cells. Science 1994: 265: 808–811.
22. Ayala A, Wang P, Ba Z F et al. Differential alterations in plasma IL-6 and TNF levels after trauma and haemorrhage. Am J Physiol 1991; 260: R167–R171.
23. Faist E, Storck M, Hultner L et al. Functional analysis of monocyte activity through synthesis patterns of pro-inflammatory cytokines and neopterin in patients in surgical intensive care. Surgery 1992; 112: 562–572.
24. Murata A, Ogawa M, Yasuda T et al. Serum interleukin-6, C-reactive protein and pancreatic secretory trypsin inhibitor (PSTI) as acute phase reactants after major thoraco-

abdominal surgery. Immunol Invest 1990; 19: 271–278.

25. Guice K S, Oldham K T, Remick D G et al. Anti-tumour necrosis factor antibody augments edema formation in caerulein-induced acute pancreatitis. J Surg Res 1991; 51: 495–499.

26. Leser H-G, Gross V, Scheibenbogen C et al. Elevation of serum interleukin-6 precedes acute phase response and reflects severity in acute pancreatitis. Gastroenterology 1991; 101: 782–785.

27. Riche F C, Cholley B P, Panis Y H et al. Inflammatory cytokine response in patients with septic shock secondary to generalised peritonitis. Crit Care Med 2000; 28: 433–437.

28. Ayala A, Perrin M M, Meldrum D R et al. Haemorrhage induced an increase in serum TNF which is not associated with elevated levels of endotoxin. Cytokine 1990; 2: 170–174.

29. Haga Y, Beppu T, Doi K et al. Systemic inflammatory response syndrome and organ dysfunction following gastrointestinal surgery. Crit Care Med 1997; 25: 1994–2000.

30. Fanning N F, Kell M R, Shorten G D et al. Circulating granulocyte macrophage colony stimulating factor in plasma of patients with SIRS delays neutrophil apoptosis through inhibition of spontaneous reactive oxygen species generation. Shock 1999; 11: 167–174.

31. Hirshberg A, Wall Jr M J, Mattox K L. Planned re-operation for trauma: a two year experience with 124 consecutive patients. J Trauma 1994; 37: 365–369.

32. Abraham E, Wunderink R, Silverman H et al. Efficacy and safety of monoclonal antibody to human tumour necrosis factor alpha in patients with sepsis syndrome. A randomised, controlled, double-blind, multicenter clinical trial. TNF-α Mab Sepsis Study Group. JAMA 1995; 273: 934–941.

33. Echtenacher B, Falk W, Mannel D N, Krammer P H. Requirement of endogenous tumour necrosis factor/cachectin for recovery from experimental peritonitis. J Immunol 1990; 145: 3762–3766.

34. Fischer Jr C J, Dhainant J F, Opal S M et al. Sepsis study group: recombinant human interleukin receptor antagonist in the treatment of patients with sepsis syndrome. JAMA 1994; 271: 1836–1843.

35. Willats S M, Radford S, Leitermann M. Effect of the antiendotoxic agent, taurolidine, in the treatment of sepsis syndrome: a placebo-controlled, double-blind trial. Crit Care Med 1995; 23: 1033–1039.

36. Gitzelmann C A, Mendoza-Sagaon M, Talamiri M A, Ahmad S A, Pegoli Jr W, Paidas C N. Cell mediated immune response is better preserved by laparoscopy than laparotomy. Surgery 2000; 127: 65–71.

37. Kehlet H. Surgical stress response: does endoscopic surgery confer an advantage? World J Surg 1999; 23: 801–807.

Philip Conaghan   Celia L. Ingham Clark

CHAPTER

3

The organisation of day surgery

The organisation of day surgery has only really become common place in the last 15 years despite its advantages, which have been mooted since the early 20th century. Nicholls reported his first series of day case patients in 1909 in the *British Medical Journal*.[1] He operated on 9000 children as day cases, half under 3 years of age, and advocated that more surgeons should do the same. However, the potential for day surgery in the modern NHS was not embraced until the publication of the first edition of the *Guidelines for Day Case Surgery* in 1985 by The Royal College of Surgeons of England. The formation of the British Association of Day Surgery in 1989 added further to the important role day surgery was to play in future provision of surgical services.

Measuring the volume of day surgery performed in individual hospitals has proved surprisingly difficult. Variation in the definition of what procedures are classified as 'day cases' and the use of day case to in-patient ratios rather than absolute numbers to measure how much day surgery is performed has led to the artificial inflation of day surgery figures for a number of centres.

The Royal College of Surgeons of England defined a surgical day case patient as one 'who is admitted for investigation or operation on a planned non-resident basis and who nonetheless requires facilities for recovery'.[2] This definition excludes upper and lower GI endoscopies, out-patient procedures such as flexible cystoscopy, and minor superficial surgery under local anaesthetic, none of which require full day case facilities for recovery. At the other extreme, patients undergoing '23-hour' or short-stay surgery are admitted as resident patients and likewise do not strictly qualify. An increasing proportion of patients treated as day cases has been encouraging (Table 3.1), but these averages hide a considerable range, with some hospitals doing minimal day surgery. In 1995, 19% of hospitals still had no day unit. Even modest improvements in these

Mr Philip Conaghan BA MRCS, Surgical Registrar, Department of General Surgery, Northampton General Hospital, NN1 5BD, UK
Mrs C.L. Ingham Clark, MChir FRCS, Consultant General Surgeon, Whittington Hospital, Highgate Hill, London N19 5NF, UK (for correspondence)

Table 3.1 Day case surgery as a percentage of the total elective surgical admissions and as absolute numbers in the UK

	% of cases	Absolute numbers (x 10^6)
1989–90	34	1.1
1993–94	48	2.1
1998–99	60	3.5

centres would lead to a marked increase in the overall average. Improvements in surgical and anaesthetic techniques will also increase the volume of day surgery performed, allowing a wider variety of procedures to be performed and reducing the morbidity of day surgery. Minimal access techniques and general anaesthetics designed to reduce postoperative nausea and vomiting have demonstrated this.

Table 3.2 Potential advantages of day surgery

Advantages to the patient	Advantages to purchaser/hospital
Pre-booked date and less likely to be cancelled	Reduced cost
Shorter waiting lists	High patient satisfaction
Easier domestic arrangements	
Earlier mobilisation	
Earlier return to normal environment	
Reduced risk of cross infection	
Avoidance of disruptive nights on hospital wards	
Less time of work	
Less psychological disturbance in children	

ADVANTAGES OF DAY SURGERY

One of the biggest obstacles to the future growth of day surgery is a failure to recognise its benefits. The potential advantages of day case surgery over inpatient treatment are listed in Table 3.2. The two considerable advantages pointed out by the Audit Commission in 1990[3] were: (i) the service offered to patients was better suited to their needs and these patients waited less time due to the fact that the increased throughput allowed more patients to be treated per list; and (ii) hospital costs are lowered and this is not offset by an increased community budget requirement.

Key point 1

- One of the biggest obstacles to the future growth of day surgery is a failure to recognise its benefits.

These advantages are not at the cost of surgical standards – the complication rate for day surgery procedures is not increased. The removal of day case patients from in-patient lists also makes available places for those that require in-patient treatment. As a result, day surgery is endorsed by The Royal College of Surgeons of England, by purchasers and providers of healthcare and by patient organisations. Surveys show a high level of patient satisfaction won by fixed date surgery given at the time of the out-patient appointment, the reduced risk of cancellation and the benefits of an early return home.

PRE-OPERATIVE SCREENING

The efficient organisation of day surgery, on which such advantages rely, is dependent on a number of factors, but none more so than appropriate patient selection. Where this system breaks down, it results in increases in admissions from the unit, complications and re-admissions. A lack of confidence follows and day surgery becomes unpopular amongst surgical consultants. Most units have countered poor selection by setting up formal pre-operative screening of referrals requiring a general anaesthetic. This is normally carried out by senior day surgery unit (DSU) nurses who use medical and social questionnaires to detect problems. Uncertainties can be discussed with anaesthetists responsible for that particular list. Such pre-operative visits also allow relevant investigations and have been encouraged in paediatric surgery to allow the children to familiarise themselves with the unit and staff prior to admission. Inappropriate referrals can also be reduced by clearly displaying the health and social criteria (Table 3.3) and procedures considered appropriate for day surgery, in surgical out-patient clinics and also sending these to GPs where direct-access theatre lists exist. A list of suitable procedures was proposed for experienced day surgery units by the British Association of Day Surgery in their annual scientific meeting in 1999 and should serve as a target for all day units (Table 3.4).

The basket of cases offered will vary according to the experience of the surgeon, anaesthetist and unit in particular procedures. Laparoscopic cholecystectomies and mastectomies have both been performed as day cases.[4,5]

Table 3.3 Health and social criteria for day surgery

Health criteria
ASA I or II; occasionally stable III or IV, e.g. brief minimally invasive procedures
Body mass index < 30
Normal airway
No recent upper respiratory tract infections
No significant past or family history of anaesthetic problems
Less than 75 years old, physiological age being more important than chronological age
Social criteria
Responsible adult to escort home and care for 24 hours postoperatively
Easy access to a telephone
Indoor bathroom

Table 3.4 Proposed trolley of procedures

BADS Trolley of Procedures 1999

1. Groin/abdominal hernia repair (inguinal, femoral, umbilical, epigastric)
2. Excision breast lump
3. Minor anal surgery (fissure/simple fistula)
4. Varicose vein surgery (including bilateral, or long and short s aphenous one leg)
5. Circumcision (including adult)
6. Release Dupuytren's contracture
7. Carpal tunnel decompression
8. Arthroscopy (including hip and shoulder)
9. Hydrocoele excision
10. Inguinal surgery children (orchidopexy and herniotomy)
11. Tonsillectomy in children
12. Correction squint
13. Bat ears/minor plastic procedures
14. SMR
15. Reduction nasal fractures
16. Cataract extraction
17. Laparoscopy ± sterilisation
18. Termination pregnancy
19. TUR/lasar/diathermy/limited resection bladder tumours
20. Pilonidal sinus excision and closure

50% of the following should be possible as day cases

21. Laparoscopic cholecystectomy (interval appendectomy)
22. Laparoscopic herniorrhaphy
23. Thoracoscopic sympathectomy
24. Submandibular gland excision
25. Partial thyroidectomy
26. Superficial parotidectomy
27. Breast cancer wide excision with axillary clearance
28. Haemorrhoidectomy
29. Urethrotomy
30. Bladder neck incision
31. Lasar prostatectomy
32. Trans cervical resection endometrium (TCRE)
33. Eyelid surgery including tarsoplasty, blepharoplasty
34. Hallux valgus ('bunion') operations
35. Arthroscopic menisectomy
36. Arthroscopic shoulder surgery (subacromial decompression)
37. Subcutaneous mastectomy
38. Rhinoplasty
39. Dentoalveolar surgery
40. Tympanoplasty

DISCHARGE PROCEDURES

At the other end of the process, discharge procedures need to be safe and efficient. Nurse-led discharge is the ideal as it avoids the need for the surgeon or anaesthetist to finish a case or list before discharge is possible. Most units have strict written guidelines to ensure that the process maintains well-established standards of care. Any problems can be discussed with the surgeon or anaesthetist as necessary, but the large majority of patients can be discharged without consultation. This role is ideal for experienced day case nurses who can go through discharge arrangements with the patient and pass on written information.

COMMUNICATION

Effective communication is vital for day surgery to succeed. Communication between doctor / nurse and patient, between staff members and in particular with the GP and primary healthcare team must be clear and up-to-date. However, despite being the cheapest of the links in DSU organisation it is one of the commonest shortcomings and the cause of about 25% of complaints by patients alone.[6] The opportunity for passing on effective information to patients begins in the out-patient clinic, continues at the pre-operative assessment visit to the unit and is re-iterated on the day of surgery. The assessment clinics in particular are opportunities to pass on written information explaining the operation planned, the possible complications, the necessary aftercare that will be required and advice on important activities such as driving, sexual intercourse and work. Patient and carer understanding of aftercare is essential before discharge can be considered safe and since discharge is an important step in day case efficiency, information must be clear and detailed. This requires experienced day case nurses and good written information. Since patients may have had a general anaesthetic only a few hours earlier, the carer must be involved in the discussion. The information should include: (i) analgesic advice (what was given peri-operatively [e.g. local anaesthetic, rectal NSAIDs] and what has been given to take home); (ii) dressings; (iii) arrangements for follow-up both with the hospital and with the primary healthcare workers (e.g. district nurses); (iv) advice on how to assist the recovery and what symptoms to expect; and (v) contact telephone numbers for early postoperative complications.

Early contact with the GP is essential as some patients will consult their GP soon after surgery (about 3% within 24 h[7] and between 4–25% in 48 h).[8,9] Faxing day case discharge letters seems the most popular way to achieve this. Future paper-free hospitals and GP surgeries will soon rely on electronic mail for efficient communication. Arrangements with district and practice nurses must be made the same day if possible to ensure adequate follow-up of patients who need treatment the following day.

FINANCIAL BENEFITS

The attraction of day surgery to hospitals and purchasers of healthcare is based on the expected financial benefits. In the US, where financial concerns drive change in surgical provision far more rapidly than in the UK, the expansion of day surgery has been quicker and it is from North America that most of the day surgery innovation comes.

There are three main ways in which day surgery is organised within the hospital structure in Britain. The traditional way is to admit patients in the same way as other elective patients onto general surgical wards, using the same theatre suite and equipment and occasionally placing the patient on the same theatre list as standard in-patients. The only difference is the attempt to discharge the patient on the same day. The second concept is to have a dedicated day ward, preferably near the theatre suite, but again use the same theatre suite and equipment as that for elective surgery. The final option is to have a dedicated unit, known as an integrated day surgery unit, which is completely separate from the other surgical suites. It is self-contained with its own ward, theatres, staff, equipment and changing rooms. It should be near the car park to prevent patients having to walk long distances postoperatively, well sign-posted and designed solely for the needs of day surgery patients. It is run as a separate department within the hospital with its own budget. The integrated DSU has become the gold standard for day units in Britain because it allows the benefits of day surgery to realise their full potential. About half of the hospitals in the UK had integrated DSUs in 1995. Treating day surgery patients on general surgical wards loses most of these benefits. For example, the nurses are not working solely with day patients and the greater needs of the in-patient elective and emergency patients take priority. Nurse-led discharge is often not possible, the ward is not in close proximity to the theatre suite and hence rapid turn around of patients is not possible and the ward cannot be locked, unlit, unheated and unstaffed in the evenings and at weekends. Beds are used for emergencies and so day case patients, like elective in-patients are cancelled as a result. The implications for patients and hospitals are considerable. The dedicated day ward solves most of these problems if situated near the theatre suite, but the use of the main theatre suite means that the unit cannot be entirely shut-down after hours and the theatre staff are not concerned with the needs of day case patients only. The integrated DSU has a dedicated nursing staff who are often able to undertake both ward and theatre duties which adds flexibility to the unit staff management. The well-practised routine of day surgery works best in this type of environment. This exacts maximum benefit for staff as well as for patients and the hospital. The extension of this concept with the development of free-standing units (FSUs) will be discussed below.

Key point 3

- The integrated day surgery unit has become the gold standard for day units in the UK because it allows the benefits of day surgery to realise their full potential.

IMPROVING EFFICIENCY

Even in hospitals with integrated DSUs there may be room to improve the efficiency of the system. The problem of non-attendance wasting valuable theatre time still persists. Ways of minimising the percentage of non-attenders include telephone reminders, letters requiring patients to confirm their theatre date up to 2 weeks before and pre-admission visits close to the date of surgery, all of which have been shown to increase compliance. When scheduled for up to 3 weeks prior to surgery, the latter significantly reduces the non-attendance rate on the day of surgery.[10] It also allows further information to be given to the patient regarding their particular operation. Patients not attending the assessment without reason are removed from the waiting list. Obviously, local anaesthetic cases do not require such screening but pre-operative letters requiring patients to confirm their appointment again improves attendance.

Those spaces that are vacant – by non-attenders or by under-booking of a list – can occasionally be filled with other suitable candidates. Figueira et al. described a system in which emergency patients with conditions and health and social profiles suitable for day surgery can be allocated vacant places at short notice provided a suitable co-ordinator is available for the task.[11]

Some surgeons consider the out-patient visit unnecessary for minor surgical procedures. 'Direct access' theatre lists allow GPs to book cases directly onto day lists. The pre-operative assessment is arranged as usual where necessary. The surgeon sees the patient for the first time on the day of surgery. This reduces out-patient lists and waiting times as shown by Gandy in a controlled trial.[12] The system runs the risk of late patient cancellation if the surgeon deems the operation inappropriate but, with patients aware of this possibility, it works well. For general anaesthetic cases, GPs must be aware of the health and social criteria of the unit. Gandy showed that 94% of those referred by the direct access route had a correct diagnosis.

Restricting the use of the day unit to those who need day surgery also improves efficiency and through-put. Procedures not requiring full day case facilities such as OGD, colonoscopy, flexible cystoscopy and minor local anaesthetic cases should be done in appropriate units where possible. The problem of under- or over-booking of lists can be a problem, especially where the lists are compiled by junior or administrative staff. Cole and Hislop[13] suggested allocating a grade, representing expected operating time, to each procedure in the day case basket for a given consultant. Theatre lists were compiled so that the sum total of grades reached a given total. By this method, they reduced time-related cancellations and the amount of wasted time per list.

EXTENDING THE CONCEPT

EXTENDED DAY SURGERY

For an efficient integrated DSU some have suggested that the standard 12 h day unit has reached its limits of development. However, the principles involved in day surgery could usefully be applied to surgery involving one overnight stay. This would open up the efficiency of the day surgery system to a wider range of cases – so-called 23 h surgery or extended day surgery. Those unhappy about performing laparoscopic cholecystectomies, thyroidectomies or mastectomies as day cases for example, may welcome a ward in which patients were admitted on the day of surgery as for day cases and discharged the following day if appropriate by day case nurses. The day unit theatres could be used with a separate overnight ward for these patients. The day case

Key point 4

- The principles involved in day surgery could usefully be applied to surgery involving one overnight stay. This would open up the efficiency of the day surgery system to a wider range of cases – so-called 23 h surgery or extended day surgery.

health and social criteria would apply although could be modified. Phillips et al.[14] demonstrated successful treatment of 354 patients in this way, allowing 77.5% of their total elective load to be treated as day case or extended day case patients. The appropriate ward could be ring-fenced to prevent it being used by emergency patients.

HOSPITAL HOTELS

Another method of extending the day case concept has been the introduction of 'hospital hotels'.[15] These are typically separate buildings adjacent to the hospital which provide accommodation for patients who are mobile and self-caring, but who require an overnight stay in hospital, often for social reasons. There are auxiliary nurses or even non-medical personnel on-site to act as the responsible adult required by the patients. Such a building only requires staffing for part of the day, can be closed for most of the weekend and hence requires less intensive staffing than a ward. Consequently, the number of potential day surgery patients increases. Such facilities are in frequent use in the US.

The 'hospital at home' concept provides whatever nursing care is required in the patient's home, hence allowing discharge the same day. This would allow the DSU to treat those previously excluded on social criteria or who required hospital admission for specialist nursing. Physiotherapists, nurses and other professionals could visit the patient's home to provide this care with access to medical care via the GP or a specialist out-reach day surgery nurse in the first instance. The latter may alleviate the concerns of some in primary care who feel that increases in the volume of day surgery would impact directly on the primary care teams. Primary care groups may wish to adopt this idea to free-up more capacity in the hospital for treating patients requiring more major surgery and reducing the waiting time for more minor surgery.

FREE STANDING UNITS

The efficiency of the integrated DSU has led to many to advocate 'free-standing units'. These are day hospitals, separate form any acute medical facility, which specialise in day surgery and investigation. The entire unit shuts down out of hours as for integrated DSUs. There are, however, obvious concerns. The lack of proximity to the main hospital is not ideal should significant complications arise. Even the steady 1% of patients requiring admission from day units would present a frequent problem for the unit. However they are extremely popular in the US and have apparently increased the efficiency of day surgery.[16] We await statistics from the few FSUs in this country (e.g. Cambridge and Epsom) The Epsom unit, owned and run by a primary medical services practice, is free to contract out to trusts for surgical and anaesthetic staff with considerable advantages for local patients (e.g. reduced waiting time, proximity of the unit [Dr T. Richardson, Medical Director, Epsom Day Surgery Unit, personal communication]). This also raises the question of who will be providing FSU facilities in the future if hospital trusts are slow to adopt such ideas.

Key point 5

- The efficiency of the integrated day surgery unit has led many to advocate 'free-standing units'. These are day hospitals, separate from any acute medical facility, which specialise in day surgery and investigation.

ADVICE LINES

The development of advice lines for day surgery patients has increased confidence in the service and should replace the practice of contacting junior surgical staff with no knowledge of the patient or the day surgery system. Instead, specialist day surgery nurses can be contacted via the hospital switchboard.

PERSONNEL AND MANAGEMENT

An efficient day case unit requires a well-structured management team. The clinical director should assume overall responsibility and should be either a consultant surgeon or anaesthetist. They are not only in a position to understand the needs of the unit but can understand and act on concerns of his/her colleagues and the nursing staff. The director should also oversee education and training within the unit. If these extra responsibilities are allocated in this way, there must be an agreement between director and Trust to reduce other hospital commitments for the director. The nurse manager is responsible for the day-to-day running of the unit, management of the nursing staff, equipment maintenance and allocation and the smooth running of theatre lists. More units now employ a business manager, especially integrated DSUs. The more independent the unit, the more vital it is to have a manager who is trained to run a business and not to rely on medical staff to carry out a second full-time job for which they were never trained.

Key point 6

- An efficient day case unit requires a well-structured management team. The clinical director should assume overall responsibility and should be either a consultant surgeon or anaesthetist.

TRAINING, AUDIT AND RESEARCH

The increasing volume of elective work carried out as day cases and the increasing demands for structured teaching programmes from medical schools, through basic surgical training and into higher surgical training, means that day surgery units cannot be organised purely with efficiency in mind. Education at all levels must be a primary concern. Many routine surgical procedures have been removed from in-patient lists and hence are unavailable for teaching in pre-operative examination, operative principles and postoperative follow-up unless teaching is a priority in day surgery units. The long-term effects of neglecting education in day surgery will be inadequately trained surgeons and doctors in general. Time must be given to surgical trainees within the structure of the day case lists. This can be achieved in a number of ways. An occasional 'trainees list', with cases tailored to the needs of a particular trainee, could be instituted – lighter than a normal list, but with direct consultant supervision. An alternative is to have one case per list which is targeted for the trainee. More elaborate plans for training have been suggested.[17] For medical students, a daily pre- and postoperative ward round carried out by a member of the firm would provide excellent exposure to common surgical problems, develop skills in history-taking and examination and gain knowledge in the principles of surgical procedures all condensed into a single session.

As with all other fields of medicine, day surgery must be active in audit and research if it is to develop and maximise its potential. Modern databases make data collection for such projects considerably easier and trainees and students should be encouraged to participate. The involvement of students has been shown to be of mutual benefit of both students and unit.[18] Patient satisfaction assessments should also be central to the day case ethos. Encouraging feedback not only provides pointers to where improvement is necessary but is known to reduce formal complaints. The Audit Commission set out ways in which this may be achieved in their document on patients' views of day surgery.[7]

Key point 7

- Many routine surgical procedures have been removed from in-patient lists and hence are unavailable for teaching in pre-operative examination, operative principles and postoperative follow-up unless teaching is a priority in day surgery units. The long-term effects of neglecting education in day surgery will be inadequately trained surgeons and doctors in general.

Much of the audit and research carried out by day case units rely on information from the community. The mutual co-operation in these matters for the benefit of the patients should encourage firm links and regular dialogue between day surgery units and primary care. Research and audit planned and executed by joint parties should be encouraged if we are determined to learn from these exercises.

CONCLUSIONS

Day surgery is now well established in the large majority of hospitals in the UK. Its success means that it will continue to expand and the improvements in surgical and anaesthetic techniques will ensure that this is possible. The increase of free-standing units will not be long in coming judging by their success in the US and this together with other initiatives will require alterations in the way we work, teach and train as surgeons.

Key points for clinical practice

- One of the biggest obstacles to the future growth of day surgery is a failure to recognise its benefits.

- The efficient organisation of day surgery is dependent on a number of factors, but none more so than appropriate patient selection.

- The integrated day surgery unit has become the gold standard for day units in the UK because it allows the benefits of day surgery to realise their full potential.

- The principles involved in day surgery could usefully be applied to surgery involving one overnight stay. This would open up the efficiency of the day surgery system to a wider range of cases – so-called 23 h surgery or extended day surgery.

- The efficiency of the integrated day surgery unit has led many to advocate 'free-standing units'. These are day hospitals, separate from any acute medical facility, which specialise in day surgery and investigation.

- An efficient day case unit requires a well-structured management team. The clinical director should assume overall responsibility and should be either a consultant surgeon or anaesthetist.

- Many routine surgical procedures have been removed from in-patient lists and hence are unavailable for teaching in pre-operative examination, operative principles and postoperative follow-up unless teaching is a priority in day surgery units. The long-term effects of neglecting education in day surgery will be inadequately trained surgeons and doctors in general.

References

1. Nicholls J. The surgery of infancy. BMJ 1909; ii: 753–754.
2. The Royal College of Surgeons of England. Commission on the Provision of Surgical Services. Report of the Working Party on Guidelines for Day Case Surgery. London: The Royal College of Surgeons of England, 1992.
3. Audit Commission. A Short Cut to Better Services. Day Surgery in England and Wales. London: HMSO, 1990.
4. Keulemans Y, Eshuis J, de-Haes H, de-Wit LT, Gouma DJ. Laparoscopic cholecystectomy: day case versus clinical observation. Ann Surg 1998; 228: 734–740.

5. Warren JL, Riley GF, Potosky AL, Klabunde CN, Richter E, Ballard-Barbash R. Trends and outcomes of outpatient mastectomy in elderly women. J Natl Cancer Inst 1998; 90: 833–840.

6. Audit Commission. Measuring Quality: The Patient's View of Day Surgery. London: HMSO, 1991.

7. Kong KL, Child DL, Donovan IA, Nasmyth-Miller D. Demand on primary healthcare after day surgery. Ann R Coll Surg Engl 1997; 79: 291–295.

8. Fletcher J, Dawes M, McWilliams J, Millar J, Griffiths S. Community health services workload: a descriptive study. Br J Gen Pract 1996; 46: 477–478.

9. Ghosh S, Sallam S. Patient satisfaction and postoperative demands on hospital and community services after day surgery. Br J Surg 1994; 81: 1635–1638.

10. Pain S, Maguire D, Leaky M, Wooler D, Ingham Clark CL. A mechanism for reducing patient non-attendance rates for day surgery. Amb Surg 1997; 5: 93–94.

11. Figueira E, Francis D, Ingham Clark CL. The introduction of emergency day surgery [abstract]. J One Day Surg 1999; 9: 4–5.

12. Gandy R. Direct access surgery [abstract]. J One Day Surg 1998; 7: 11.

13. Cole BD, Hislop WS. A grading system in day surgery. Effective utilisation of theatre time. J R Coll Surg Edinb 1998; 43: 87–88.

14. Phillips D, Healey J, McWhinnie D, Caballero C, Souter R. Extended day surgery. J One Day Surg 1999; 8: 5–6

15. Jarrett MED, Wallace M, Jarrett PEM. The benefits of a hospital hotel in ambulatory surgery. Abstracts of the First International Congress on Ambulatory Surgery, Brussels No 13, 1995.

16. Gallinat A, Nugent W, Lueken RP, Moller CP, Busche D. Gynaecological laparoscopy and hysteroscopy in a day clinic: trends and perspectives. J Am Assoc Gynecol Laparosc 1994; 1: 103–110.

17. Sharp RJ, Wellwood J. The training implications of day case surgery. Br J Hosp Med 1996; 55: 472–475.

18. Rudkin GE, O'Driscoll MCE, Limb R. Can medical students contribute to quality assurance programmes in day surgery? Med Educ 1999; 33: 509–514.

David J. Wheatley

Clinical governance and setting standards in surgery

To surgeons, advances in surgery would suggest new interventions, new technology, new drugs, or better understanding of pathophysiology. However, for the general public, surgical advances mean little unless they translate into widely accessible and effective treatment available within the National Health Service (NHS). Delivery of the highest possible quality of surgical care to all would be no less an advance in surgery than many of the currently emerging surgical technologies. Seen in this light, the concepts embodied in clinical governance offer promise of advancing the standards of surgery in the UK and are, therefore, relevant to all surgeons.

The concept of clinical governance has been introduced to put emphasis on quality of clinical care at the forefront of all NHS activity. Setting of standards and monitoring of clinical performance will be central to clinical governance. Surgeons may find some of the required adjustments uncomfortable. Cardiac surgeons have for some time been particularly exposed to similar pressures to those which have prompted the introduction of clinical governance.[1] Their experience has relevance to other surgical specialties, and some recommendations are possible for those contemplating the new challenges of clinical governance.

The UK NHS circular HSC 1999/065 of 16 March 1999 has been widely circulated and gives guidance on implementation of clinical governance.[2] Clinical governance is seen as 'a framework through which NHS organisations are accountable for continuously improving the quality of their services and safeguarding high standards of care by creating an environment in which excellence in clinical care will flourish'. Teamwork, partnership and communication are emphasised.

Quality of clinical care will encompass evidence-based medicine, effective audit, and cost-effectiveness in clinical care.[2] Clinical governance goes further to include modernisation of hospitals and equipment, provision of sufficient and

Prof. David J. Wheatley MD ChM FRCS FRCP, Department of Cardiac Surgery, Royal Infirmary, Queen Elizabeth Building, 10 Alexandra Parade, Glasgow G31 2ER, UK

appropriately trained staff, and resources to meet clinical needs throughout the NHS in a convenient, prompt and efficient way.[2–4] The injection of political will on the ambitious scale envisaged in clinical governance coincides with widespread public concern about well recognised inadequacies in the NHS.

WHAT IS THE RELEVANCE OF CLINICAL GOVERNANCE TO SURGERY?

Improving health and ensuring easy access for all to the highest possible quality of medical care are such obviously desirable goals that all in the NHS would wish to commit themselves to the concepts of clinical governance. Moreover, future funding will be dependent on demonstration of success of such commitment.

Most surgeons feel instinctively that delivery of high quality care to patients is fundamental to their activity. To see this promulgated through the 'new' concept of clinical governance, as though clinicians had not given any thought to quality of care in the past, risks causing offence and disillusionment. Nevertheless, as a concept for the entire NHS, and as a counterbalance to the recent emphasis on cost containment and cost justification, the new moves should be welcomed.

The requirement for standards of clinical quality to be a responsibility of hospital chief executives inevitably means that others will scrutinize the work of surgeons, and will make demands on surgical activity in new ways and with new-found authority.[5] Surgeons must, therefore, be prepared to adapt to shared opinion and authority in areas they might consider exclusively their own.

The need for adequate resources, staff and facilities is not unique to surgery, but surgeons often identify these as being limitations on their ability to provide quality care. The opportunity offered by clinical governance for surgeons to correlate quality of surgical care with provision of resources, staffing and facilities will allow them to identify and rectify shortcomings with greater chance of success than in the past.

The principles of monitoring activity, setting standards, auditing outcomes and modifying clinical practice in the light of outcome, with teamwork and adherence to management protocols, integrated care pathways or guidelines embracing the concepts of evidence based medicine apply to all specialties.[6–8] However, surgery imposes demands not matched in other disciplines to anywhere near the same extent.

IN THE CONTEXT OF CLINICAL GOVERNANCE, WHY MAY SURGERY DIFFER FROM OTHER SPECIALTIES?

The surgeon's individual professional performance can be related to clinical outcome with an immediacy and accountability unmatched by most other health professionals

Death on an operating table is perhaps the most obvious and dramatic adverse clinical outcome, and is invariably perceived as the 'responsibility of the surgeon'. It is not a big leap of imagination to see this becoming the 'fault of the surgeon'. Surgeons can easily be made to feel unfairly scrutinised and criticised, or be made the scapegoat for inadequacies elsewhere in the totality of clinical care.

The conduct of a surgical operation is largely the responsibility of the individual surgeon and frequently cannot be a team effort

Teamwork is a feature of clinical governance. Many aspects of operations, such as the judgement about where to make a resection line, the skill in sewing abnormal tissues, and the speed and accuracy with which technical manoeuvres are accomplished, may have a profound influence on outcome. However, these are issues that are difficult to share with a 'team'.

Variability in patient characteristics, such as co-morbidity, anatomical variants and nature of pathology, play a more important role in outcome for surgical management than they may in other, non-invasive management strategies in medicine

Anatomical variants, and the location, nature and extent of pathology may all influence surgical outcome in a profound manner. Add to this the variability in patients' ability to withstand operation as a result of age, nutritional status, pulmonary function, coronary disease, renal function and co-morbidity, and it is easy to appreciate the difficulty in comparing outcomes for surgery between surgeons or surgical units. Although surgeons appreciate the influence of these factors, others may not. Surgeons risk being perceived as unduly defensive of their own performance if claims of clinical variability in patients are thought to obscure critical assessment of the surgeon's own role in outcome.

In addition to the necessary theoretical knowledge base, the surgeon has a requirement for practical skills not required of many other medical professionals

Surgeons rightly emphasise the need for comprehensive knowledge of the diseases they treat, and many disdain the concept of being regarded as merely a 'technician'. Yet herein lies a danger of underplaying the importance and uniqueness of the surgeon's role in the operating room. Surgeons must take a prominent role in clinical governance precisely because others are unlikely to fully understand the practical skill base in surgery.

Concentration on current practice and outcome may inhibit innovation and progress into new fields and techniques

Though this is a concern sometimes expressed, it is not unique to surgery. However, surgeons in the past have often had an individual pioneering role, the nature of which would not find an easy place in the setting of clinical governance.

> **Key point 1**
>
> - Surgeons should take the opportunities for local involvement in clinical governance.

WHAT HAS BEEN THE EXPERIENCE IN CARDIAC SURGERY?

The changes in public and political perception of medical practice experienced in cardiac surgery, in the UK, the US and elsewhere, have relevance to many of the proposals in clinical governance.

There has long been a wealth of detailed information about outcome and recommended techniques for coronary surgery, generated from leading academic medical centres, often bearing the imprimatur of the most respected surgical authorities in the world. However, in recent years, the high cost and the sheer scale of coronary surgical practice have made it vulnerable to more sceptical public and health management organisation attention. Much of this attention has focused on cost concerns, but surgical mortality has also made it a target for detailed public scrutiny, with the implied aim of curtailing poor practice and encouraging the best. The most high profile examples of this scrutiny are from the states of Pennsylvania and New York,[9,10] which have for several years published the operative mortality for each individual cardiac surgeon in these states, together with numbers of operations undertaken, and estimates of expected mortality, based on patient characteristics, for each surgeon. Anaesthetists, cardiologists, nurses and managers do not feature in these publications. The vulnerability of the individual surgeon, the absence of the team concept when under scrutiny, and the need for comparable outcome measures, risk stratification and standards are obvious.

The fact that traditional gathering of data, reporting of outcomes and setting of standards by cardiac surgeons, even when of exemplary standard, has been unable to adequately meet the demands of the public and health care administrators in the US has important lessons for surgery in the UK. Independent and public scrutiny is inevitable.

HOW HAVE CARDIAC SURGEONS RESPONDED?

A number of strategies had already been adopted in cardiac surgery with the aim of improving practice. These proved inadequate to shelter the specialty from criticism, and some even argue that they drew attention, making unwelcome scrutiny easier.[1] The moves have since been expanded with the aim of helping surgeons to adapt to the new ethos in which they work.

Documentation of outcome for surgical procedures and development of risk stratification to allow prediction of outcome

The UK National Cardiac Surgical Register, established in 1979 by the UK Society of Cardiothoracic Surgeons, required submission of numbers and types of operations in cardiac surgical units on a voluntary basis, with unit-specific, rather than surgeon-specific, outcome. Though innovative at its inception, lack of external validation of data, difficulties in achieving complete submissions from all units, anxieties over confidentiality, and the limited nature of the data have been problems.[1]

In the US, the Society of Thoracic Surgeons established a database for cardiac surgery in 1989. When the 1998 figures are in there will be over 1,340,000 procedures in the database making it possible to refine further accurate risk stratification for surgical outcome for the common adult cardiac surgical procedures.[11] Work is in hand to establish similar databases for General Thoracic Surgery and for Congenital Heart Surgery. Together with the already well established Heart and Heart/Lung Transplant Registry, these databases will cover the majority of all surgical procedures in cardiothoracic surgery in the US. Additionally, there are regional databases such as that of the Northern New England regional group.[12]

The UK Society of Cardiothoracic Surgeons has encouraged development of a detailed database with independent validation, with the aim of refining risk stratification specifically for UK practice.[1] The widely applied Parsonnet scoring system is now being challenged by other systems for greater precision in predicting operative risk for cardiac surgery.[13–15] A further feature of databases in cardiothoracic surgery is the move towards international standardisation.

Databases have given cardiac surgeons world-wide authoritative information on outcome by which to judge their own practice, providing a strong personal incentive to quality of care. The Northern New England regional group have shown that its database has facilitated improved quality of coronary surgical care.[12] In allowing establishment of systems for risk stratification, they have enabled individual surgical outcomes to be more fairly compared. Contribution to a database provides a powerful defence against criticism of defensive attitudes over outcome. Use of databases has also established the value of certain surgical practices, for example the use of the internal mammary artery as a preferred coronary bypass conduit, spawning efforts to increase the use of arterial conduits.[11]

Establishment of accurate databases is an inherent part of clinical governance. The time, personnel and resources required for developing and maintaining such databases are considerable, involving computing and software development, centralised data management and local input managers in hospitals. Other surgical specialties may be less easy to document because of their diverse nature, and mortality may not be a satisfactory outcome measure.[16,17] Even in cardiac surgery, mortality is far from the most appropriate outcome measure. Long-term angina relief, survival benefit and reduction in cardiac events are much more relevant to the majority of patients, and may be determined in considerable measure by surgical performance, but their documentation is time-consuming and difficult to the point of being impractical as an outcome measure applicable to all surgeons.

Establishment of practice guidelines

The sheer volume of literature on clinical practice makes it virtually impossible for most surgeons to stay up-to-date. One way of overcoming this difficulty is the use of clinical guidelines. In cardiac surgery there are guidelines to many aspects of practice, prepared by those most knowledgeable and active in the specialty. Not only would familiarity with guidelines help to keep surgeons up-to-date, but adherence to guidelines would insulate surgeons from adverse criticism of their work.

The American College of Cardiology and the American Heart Association have produced management guidelines for many aspects of heart diseases, including the surgical treatment of coronary disease.[18] The European Society of Cardiology has similarly produced guidelines for management of many cardiovascular conditions.

Setting standards

In cardiac surgery, operative mortality is the most immediate and verifiable outcome measure which gives an indication of surgical standards, provided that risk stratification is applied. The UK Society of Cardiothoracic Surgeons requires documentation of operative mortality for all UK cardiac surgeons for elective, first time coronary bypass surgery.[1] Although an upper limit for mortality is not defined, outliers can readily be identified, and followed up for further detail or investigation as appropriate. Beyond consideration of mortality, little has been done to set standards based on outcome for cardiac surgery.

Key point 2

- National specialty associations and groups must have an important role.

WHAT RECOMMENDATIONS CAN BE MADE FOR SURGERY IN FACING THE CHALLENGES OF CLINICAL GOVERNANCE?

Although much of the literature on clinical governance emphasises local action at Trust hospital level,[7] it is inconceivable that each surgical unit could establish meaningful databases, define risks, set standards and guidelines, and monitor outcomes without reference to what is happening in the wider surgical world. International and national databases and guidelines must have a major role. Many up-to-date and highly authoritative guidelines exist for management of most of the common conditions encountered throughout surgical practice and many surgeons have long been well familiar with such guidelines. In common with cardiac surgeons, many in other surgical specialties will feel that their practice is already ahead of clinical governance. Centrally funded national audits, such as the UK *National Confidential Enquiry into Peri-operative Deaths* already fulfil many of the functions envisaged in clinical governance.[7]

Key point 3

- Existing databases will need expansion; new databases may be needed.

Documentation of outcome

Accurate record keeping, with documentation of relevant patient characteristics, surgical procedures, complications or mortality should be the responsibility of all surgeons and is a pre-requisite for clinical governance. Standardised methods for collection of such data, together with regular, formal review of outcome within a unit, make for better compliance and should act as a spur to better quality and identify specific problems of a unit or an individual surgeon.

Risk stratification should be possible for the commoner surgical procedures, but this requires large databases, which must be the responsibility of a professional society or grouping with the authority to collect and verify data on an appropriate scale.[16,17]

Key point 4

- Risk stratification should be developed to allow fair comparison of outcome.

Mortality will not be a useful outcome measure for many procedures and each specialty will have to identify appropriate outcome measures for itself. Recurrence of hernia, recurrence of tumour, need for revision arthroplasty, or rates of surgical infection are but a few examples of outcomes which may be more clinically meaningful, depending on the specialty. Each of these outcomes is more difficult and time-consuming to evaluate, and the results are not as immediately applicable as is mortality. There is a risk that clinical governance will focus attention on short-term, easily observed complications, rather than more clinically appropriate, long-term outcome measures. A few, relatively simple outcome measures will need to be chosen for general use by the professional organisations of each specialty in order to allow any meaningful comparisons nationally and internationally. This does not preclude local initiatives to tackle specific problems, such as outbreaks of wound infection, or excessive use of blood products.

Establishment of practice guidelines

Demonstration that a surgical unit is following authoritative practice guidelines is a convincing way of showing its commitment to quality of clinical care. Many guidelines exist. The National Institute for Clinical Excellence will join established bodies such as professional surgical organisations, the Cochrane Collaboration, and the Scottish Intercollegiate Guidelines Network to give highly authoritative and up-to-date guidelines which could not be matched on an individual unit or Trust hospital level.[7]

Key point 5

- Nationally recognised clinical guidelines should be adopted.

Setting standards

It is intended that the NHS Performance Assessment Framework will set 'high level performance indicators' across medicine, and clinical indicators such as mortality, or re-admission following hip replacement are mentioned as examples.[2] Setting of standards must be based on knowledge of existing outcomes, and must be applied to procedures which are done in large numbers by a substantial proportion of the surgical specialty. Thus, operations such as hip replacement, resection for colon cancer, or resection of abdominal aortic aneurysm may be amenable to such scrutiny. This is where national professional specialty organisations must be active in ensuring that clinically relevant standards are chosen, that comparability between centres can be assured, and that care is taken in interpreting results.

The measures advocated above will not alone solve all problems for surgeons adapting to the needs of clinical governance, but they would go a long way. In addition, the need for sharing responsibility throughout a surgical career inevitably raises the issue of teamwork in surgery. A team work approach is envisaged within the concept of clinical governance, with care pathways having a prominent role. In the era of Calman training and the European Time Directive previous dependence of surgeons on a junior staffing structure to undertake peri-operative management is no longer possible. In this respect, a greater reliance on teams including well-trained nursing staff, following care pathways, is necessary and should enhance total surgical care.[8] Teamwork can best be initiated by consultants working together more closely. The general encouragement of more structured life-long learning and development of surgical skills is inherent in the concept of clinical governance, and can only be to the benefit of future surgeons and patients alike.

Innovation and progress will require multidisciplinary collaboration on an increasing scale. Effective new techniques will come into general use far more quickly and safely as a result of careful, scientific evaluation than they would if advocated by enthusiasts without objective evaluation. It is of interest to note that in the US, transmyocardial laser revascularisation and 'beating heart' surgery have recently emerged in clinical practice,[19,20] and that the climate of clinical trial and outcome assessment, far from inhibiting these new surgical procedures, seems to have facilitated their acceptance. Clinical Governance is likely to enhance the chances of early and wide-spread adoption of innovative and effective techniques. There is an NHS Research and Development Programme which has the aim of stimulating research, and the National Research Register helps to promulgate this research.

Key point 6 & 7

- Relevant outcome measures must be established within each surgical specialty.
- Standards or performance indicators should be simple and clinically relevant.

SUMMARY

In summary, UK surgeons must stay in touch with political and organisational changes in the NHS and must participate in moulding opinion and implementing the changes. Although clinical governance is concerned at local Trust hospital level with improving quality of clinical care, surgeons must work through their specialist organisations to benefit most from experience of others in documenting their practice, adopting appropriate guidelines, achieving standards, and ensuring rational and orderly measures are followed to meet the aims of clinical governance and ensure that best quality surgical practice is indeed readily available to all.

Key points for clinical practice

- Surgeons should take the opportunities for local involvement in clinical governance.

- National specialty associations and groups must have an important role.

- Existing databases will need expansion; new databases may be needed.

- Risk stratification should be developed to allow fair comparison of outcome.

- Nationally recognised clinical guidelines should be adopted.

- Relevant outcome measures must be established within each surgical specialty.

- Standards or performance indicators should be simple and clinically relevant.

References

1. Keogh BE, Dussek J, Watson D, Magee P, Wheatley DJ. Public confidence and cardiac surgical outcome [editorial]. BMJ 1998; 316: 1759–1760.
2. Department of Health. Clinical Governance: Quality in the New NHS. Health Service Circular 1999/065. London: HMSO, 1999.
3. Department of Health. A First Class Service: Quality in the New NHS. London: HMSO, 1998.
4. Department of Health. The New NHS: Modern, Dependable. London: HMSO, 1997.
5. Donaldson LJ. Clinical governance: a statutory duty for quality improvement [editorial]. J Epidemiol Community Health 1998; 52: 73–74.
6. Gray TA. Clinical governance. Ann Clin Biochem 2000: 37: 9–15.
7. Lugon M, Secker-Walker J. Clinical Governance. Making it Happen. London: The Royal Society of Medicine. 1999.
8. Ellis BW, Johnson S. The care pathway: a tool to enhance clinical governance. Br J Clin Gov 1999; 4: 61–71.
9. Localio AR, Hamory BH, Fisher AC, TenHave TR. The public release of hospital and physician mortality data in Pennsylvania. A case study. Med Care 1997; 35: 272–286.
10. Hannan EL, Kilburn H, Racz M, Shields E, Chassin MR. Improving the outcomes of coronary artery bypass surgery in New York State. JAMA 1994; 271: 761–766.
11. Ferguson TB, Dziuban SW, Edwards FH et al. The STS National Database: current changes and challenges for the new millennium. Ann Thorac Surg 2000; 69: 680–691.
12. Munoz JJ, Birkmeyer NJ, Dacey LJ et al. Trends in rates of re-exploration for haemorrhage after coronary artery bypass surgery. Northern New England Cardiovascular Disease Study Group. Ann Thorac Surg 1999; 68: 943–944.
13. Parsonnet V, Dean D, Bernstein AD. A method of uniform stratification of risk for evaluating the results of surgery in acquired heart disease. Circulation 1989; 79 (Suppl 1): 3–12.

14. Jones RH, Hannan EL, Hammermeister KE et al. Identification of preoperative variables needed for risk adjustment of short-term mortality after coronary artery bypass graft surgery. J Am Coll Cardiol 1996; 28: 1478–1487.

15. Orr RK, Maini BS, Dumas FD et al. A comparison of four severity-adjusted models to predict mortality after coronary artery bypass graft surgery. Arch Surg 1995; 130: 301–306.

16. Copeland GP, Jones D, Walters M. POSSUM: a scoring system for surgical audit. Br J Surg 1991; 78: 356–360.

17. Pillai SB, van Rij AM, Williams S et al. Complexity- and risk-adjusted model for measuring surgical outcome. Br J Surg 1999; 86: 1567–1572.

18. ACC/AHA/ACP-ASIM guidelines for the management of patients with chronic stable angina: executive summary and recommendations. A report of the American College of Cardiology/American Heart Association Task Force on Practice guidelines (Committee on management of patients with chronic stable angina). Circulation 1999; 99: 2829–2848.

19. Jones JW, Schmidt SE, Richman DW et al. YAG laser transmyocardial revascularization relieves angina and improves functional status. Ann Thorac Surg 1999; 67: 1596–1601.

20. Arom KV, Flavin TF, Emery RW et al. Safety and efficacy of off-pump coronary artery bypass grafting. Ann Thorac Surg 2000; 69: 704–710.

Vardhini Vijay   Christobel Saunders

The breast cancer family history clinic

With the explosion in molecular genetics and the identification and cloning of genes responsible for many of the common cancers, there has not been a time when patients and medical professionals alike are more aware of the importance of a family history of cancer. Though the inheritance of a cancer-causing gene plays the main role in familial cancer risk, shared environmental, dietary and hormonal factors may also be important.

The percentage contribution of genetic/familial cases to the overall cancer incidence is low (5–10% in the case of breast cancer[1]). These women generally have a younger age of onset of cancer, have unique psycho-oncological problems and are amenable to screening and preventive strategies. A close study of this population may add further information about genetic-environmental interactions and, in the longer term, may facilitate cancer prevention by genetic, hormonal, dietary or environmental modulation.

Key point 1

- Though genetic/familial cases contribute to only 5–10% of breast cancer cases, a close study of cancer families may add valuable information on gene–environment actions.

Many familial cancers are inter-related and genetic mutations in a family that predispose individuals to one cancer may also predispose them to other related cancers. Though it would be ideal to have all familial cancers under one

Ms Vardhini Vijay MS DNB FRCS, Surgical Registrar, Withington Hospital, Highgate Hill, London N19 5NF, UK (for correspondence)
Ms Christobel Saunders FRCS, Associate Professor, University Department of Surgery, Royal Perth Hospital, GPO Box 2213, Perth WA 6847, Australia

umbrella in a single clinic, in reality the bulk of unaffected and at risk individuals present as 'worried well' to their GPs and are referred on to the respective specialists, with a proportion going on to see a geneticist. The authors' interest is in breast cancer and, having recently set up a breast cancer family history clinic,[2] we will now describe some of the factors that need to be considered in setting up such a clinic. Though our experience is limited to breast cancer, the principles can be applied to any familial cancer.

ARE BREAST CANCER FAMILY HISTORY CLINICS NECESSARY?

Identification of the *BRCA1* gene in 1994[3] and *BRCA2* gene in 1995[4] has heightened the interest of women with a family history of breast cancer in genetic testing. With this increased awareness has developed an over-perception of risk,[5] and there is a subtle pressure on symptomatic breast clinics to cater to a population of 'worried-well' whose anxiety is to a certain extent alleviated by regular check-ups. However, the requirements of these women cannot be catered for effectively in a symptomatic breast clinic setting. Deciding whether a woman is indeed at risk requires some specialist knowledge that may be lacking in junior staff. Knowing if, and how frequently to offer, screening requires familiarity with protocols; risk explanation and counselling takes time, which is always in short supply in a busy symptomatic clinic. Hence, there is a need for specialised family history clinics to deal with these issues allotting ample time for risk explanation, counselling and discussion.

However, identifying the need alone is not sufficient to justify the existence of specialised family cancer clinics. The ultimate goal of any programme of risk assessment, screening and preventive management is to reduce mortality and, until such a time as that can be demonstrated, family history clinics need to be necessarily research-based[6] and actively audit their activity.

Key point 2

- Until a programme of risk assessment, screening and preventative management can be demonstrated to have a favourable effect on breast cancer mortality, family history clinics need to be research-based.

SETTING UP A BREAST CANCER FAMILY HISTORY CLINIC

FUNDING

The family history clinic does not serve a population with an identified illness, and hence sits uncomfortably within the hospital structure. At the same time, it requires specialist input and thus cannot be relegated as a community health resource. Family history risk counselling is not seen as a priority by the health authorities and hence obtaining the finances to set up and run such a clinic can be difficult. It is important to emphasise the potential savings that can be made in other areas, especially the symptomatic service. If carefully researched, a business case can be made for separate funding of family history clinics from within the existing hospital budget.

A recent survey in our own clinic found that 10% of all new referrals to the breast clinic are actually 'worried well' with a family history of breast cancer. There are also a small, but significant, percentage of women within a breast out-patient clinic system, who are getting inappropriate follow-up and screening. They are usually seen by junior staff who are often not confident enough to take a decision to discharge them. Even if discharged, these highly anxious women inevitably return with further complaints as they feel much more reassured if they are seen regularly in a specialist clinic.

The structured protocols of the family history clinic will hopefully avoid screening mammography being offered inappropriately and save wastage of this resource. Furthermore, the informal setting of a family history clinic and the longer time that can be spent reassuring these women should alleviate their anxiety sufficiently to prevent their re-referral with non-specific symptoms.

STAFFING

Once funding has been organised, it is important to give consideration to the staff that will be necessary to run the clinic, and their roles.

Counselling

The mainstay of the work in a family history clinic will be counselling of women with a family history. A doctor with an interest in cancer genetics (whether a surgeon, an oncologist or a staff-grade doctor) or a genetics-trained nurse can counsel low- and moderate-risk women and provide basic information to high-risk women about genetic testing and other options. The presence of a geneticist in the clinic, though ideal for prompt counselling of high-risk women, is not necessary as long as there is easy access for referral.

Breast examination

Breast examination is often part of the initial appointment session, as some of these women have specific breast symptoms. As these women are at increased risk, it is necessary for this examination to be performed by an experienced doctor or a nurse trained in breast examination. This can be a problem, as the personnel who have been trained in genetics are not necessarily experienced in breast examination. Hence the presence or support of a breast surgeon or health personnel trained in breast examinations is required.

Clerical/database staff

Until the value of family history clinics is proven, these clinics have to be research-based. Hence management of data for future analysis is a vital part of this clinic and a database manager is an integral part of the team.

Though the database can generate most of the routine correspondence, there is sometimes the need for individualised letters to be sent out. Drawing out pedigrees prior to risk assessment and ascertainment of diagnoses in the family are also time-consuming as is maintenance of notes and responding to telephonic queries.

Staff training

Most of the above roles require special training, and it is important that appropriately trained staff are ready to take on their planned roles when the clinic starts. Sitting in on clinics that are already running gives valuable insight into day-to-day problem solving.

Key point 3

- Staff training, links with symptomatic, screening and genetic services and long-term funding should all be considered well in advance of starting a family history clinic.

ALLIED SERVICES

Integration with other services is vital to the smooth running of a family history clinic and it is important that internal referral patterns are established in advance to facilitate quick access to these services (Fig. 5.1). Another factor that needs to be determined in advance is whether follow-up will be provided at the clinic itself or by the general practitioners (GPs) or referring physicians. The advantage of follow-up within the clinic is that all data can be prospectively recorded for future analysis. However, the workload increases and if there is a mechanism in place for relaying follow-up information promptly to the clinic, then it is not necessary.

Symptomatic breast clinic

In the event of discovery of a breast lump, a fast track referral to the symptomatic breast clinic is necessary. Though the referral for imaging and

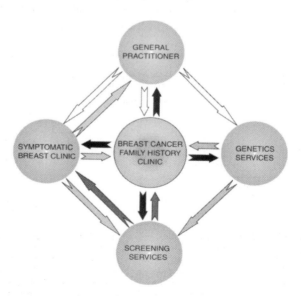

Fig. 5.1 Allied services.

fine needle aspiration if necessary can be done from the family history clinic itself, arrangements have to be in place for an appointment to the next out-patient clinic for discussion of results.

Mammographic screening

The family history clinic is not necessarily a 'one-stop' clinic, but if mammography is recommended based on the risk assessment, it has to be decided in advance whether this will be done as part of the family history clinic service or locally by the referring personnel. If performed as part of the service, links have to be built up with the screening service, so that mammography can be performed if not the same day then at least as soon as possible and the report communicated to the clinic. Funds also have to be available for long-term provision of mammographic services.

Genetics services

A genetics service is probably the most important of the alliances that a family history clinic should have. Apart from the obvious high-risk case requiring genetic counselling and testing, there are certain families that may fit into other genetic syndromes, and the occasional family where risk assessment may be difficult (Fig. 5.2). In these situations, it is helpful to have access to fairly quick advice from a geneticist as to which patients should be referred on.

REFERRALS

It is important to determine in advance protocols and referral criteria for GPs. Despite distributing these criteria widely, inappropriate referrals from GPs and surgeons do occur. These mainly take the form of women who have a very weak family history, are at no increased risk compared to the general population and hence do not require extra screening.

The possible reasons for inappropriate referrals are ignorance, lack of confidence, patient pressure or even fear of litigation. Ignorance can be tackled

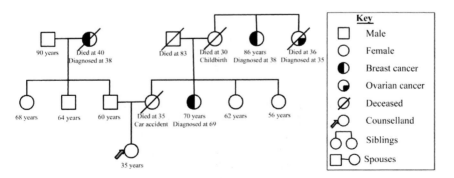

Fig. 5.2 A difficult-to-assess pedigree. The counselland's mother and maternal grandmother have died young. Though there is a strong likelihood of a genetic predisposition to breast-ovarian cancer in the maternal great-aunts, it is difficult to say if this has passed down to the counselland's mother's generation. The breast cancer in the maternal aunt could be sporadic as the age of onset is late. There is also some increased risk from the paternal side due to the young age of onset in the paternal grandmother.

Key point 4

• The family history clinic's referral criteria and management protocols should be consistent and widely circulated to general practitioners and other referrers to avoid inappropriate referrals.

by educating GPs about family history and risk. It is equally important to educate the population on what is and what is not a significant family history. Both these groups may also have an unrealistic expectation of screening in early detection. The pitfalls of screening especially in the younger age group need to be emphasised. GPs should also be confident about their own assessment of risk and the risk level at which they should refer patients. This confidence can be built by a consistency in the clinic's protocols and risk management. The referral protocol for our clinic is shown in Figure 5.3.

RISK ASSESSMENT

Many different algorithms are now available to calculate the risk of developing breast cancer. Some of these base the risk calculation on family history alone, while others use hormonal and familial factors to calculate risk. However, lack of data on relatives and early deaths of family members due to other causes before they have had a chance to develop cancer can contribute to inaccurate risk calculations. Furthermore, the interaction between environmental, hormonal and genetic factors and how this interaction impacts on risk is still unknown.

The first step in risk assessment is to draw out a pedigree like the one in Figure 5.2. This gives a good overview of the entire family and it is possible to identify if the family is a breast/ovarian cancer family or if some other related cancers are more common. Families belonging to the Li Fraumeni syndrome or hereditary non-polyposis colonic cancer syndrome can be identified in this way and referred on to the geneticist. If the family is a predominantly

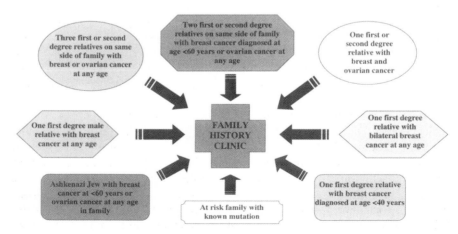

Fig. 5.3 Referral criteria.

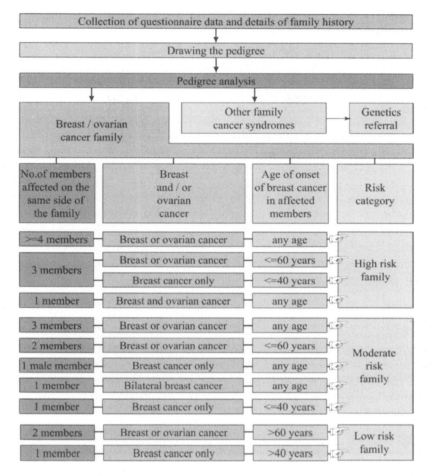

Fig. 5.4 The steps involved in risk stratification.

breast/ovarian cancer family, it is useful to mentally stratify the family into high-, moderate- or a low-risk category based on the number of members affected by breast/ovarian cancer and their ages at onset. Further assessment of numerical risk is most useful in the moderate-risk group as this contains the widest risk spectrum. The management options for the high- and low-risk categories are more clear-cut. The steps involved in risk stratification are shown in Figure 5.4.

The two main numerical risk assessment algorithms, modifications of which are used in most of the family history/genetics clinics are the Gail and the Claus models. The Gail model is based on an analysis of white women in the Breast Cancer Detection Demonstration Project who were being screened annually.[7] In this study, the factors that were shown to affect breast cancer risk were current age, age at menarche, age at first live birth, number of previous breast biopsies and number of affected first degree relatives. However, some subsequent studies have not validated the synergistic role of some of the above factors against the background of a family history.[8] The role of breast biopsies in increasing breast cancer risk outside a North American setting is also questionable.

The Claus model[9,10] is based on an analysis of the Cancer and Steroid Hormone Study dataset that includes 4730 patients with histologically confirmed breast cancer (age 20–54 years) and 4688 control subjects who were frequency matched to patients by geographic region and 5-year age intervals. The data set also includes family histories of breast cancer in mothers and sisters of both patients and control subjects. The factors used by the Claus model to calculate risk are current age, number of relatives with breast cancer and the age of onset of breast cancer in relatives. However, it takes into account only first and second degree relatives and can cater for up to 2 relatives affected by breast cancer. Hence it underestimates risk in a genetic environment and when ovarian cancer is also present in the family.

The above problems have to a certain extent been circumvented by the BRCAPRO risk calculation algorithm.[11] This uses a Bayesian method of risk calculation and takes into account breast and ovarian cancer in first and second degree relatives. The prevalence and penetrance data used can be based on the Claus dataset or the Breast Cancer Linkage Consortium data.

Key points 5 & 6

- Risk assessment involves collection of family history data, drawing out a pedigree, ascertaining that breast and ovarian cancer are the predominant cancers and stratifying the family into a high-, moderate- or low-risk category.

- Numerical risk assessment can be done using the Gail, Claus or BRCAPRO models and their modifications.

Even if the risk of being a gene carrier can be accurately calculated, there still remains the question of gene penetrance. What makes some mutation carriers develop cancer and others not? The penetrance data available in the literature are based on studies of high-risk families only and may be falsely high. A multicentre epidemiological study of BRCA mutation carriers and their families is currently underway and will hopefully give more information on genetic-environmental interactions and gene penetrance.

RISK COMMUNICATION

Once the risk has been assessed, it is then time to communicate all this information to the counselland. Studies have shown that optimum risk awareness and optimum anxiety predispose to optimum uptake of screening and preventative resources.[12] However, women who are aware and worried about their family history often over-estimate their own risk.[13,14] These pre-conceived risk perceptions usually depend upon their personal experience with the disease. Women from high risk families who have never been directly involved in the care of a relative with breast cancer or whose relatives have survived after breast cancer can be quite complacent about their risk. However,

> **Key point 7**
>
> • Women with a family history generally tend to overestimate their own risk of developing breast cancer. Even one-to-one risk counselling does not seem to have a long-term effect on an individual's personal risk perception.

if a woman has nursed her 70-year-old mother and watched her suffer from metastatic disease, it may be difficult to convince her that her own risk is low.

There is a lot of debate about what is the clearest way to explain someone's risk of developing a disease. Some women are unclear about numerical risk and may be more comfortable if their risk is categorised as high, moderate or low. However, the spectrum of moderate-risk is vast and placement of an individual woman's risk within this vast spectrum may be difficult without recourse to numerical values.

Numerical risk itself can be given in a variety of ways. One of the much-favoured methods is the **odds ratio**: 'you have a 1 in x chance of developing breast cancer'. The odds ratio should be qualified with the time period over which it is valid. The **relative risk** is another method of explaining risk: 'you are 3 times as likely to develop breast cancer as a woman without your family history'. Obviously, this requires knowledge of the baseline risk for a given age. Probably the most accurate method and also the most difficult to understand is the **absolute risk**:[15] 'you have a 20% chance of developing breast cancer...'. Again here, it needs to be qualified with the time period over which it is valid, i.e. '...before you are 79'. Even with the same relative risk, absolute risk varies with age as it also depends on mortality from other causes.[15]

Unfortunately, various studies using different individualised risk explanation methods with or without audio-visual aids have not shown any effect on risk perception or anxiety in the longer term.[5,16,17] Our clinic uses a graphical risk explanation method and initial studies on patients' perception of their own anxiety have been promising. Two graphs are shown while explaining risk – the first shows the absolute remaining lifetime risk for a

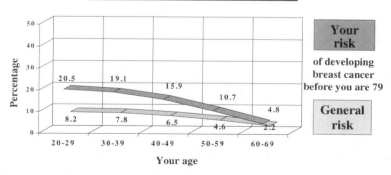

You have one 1st degree relative who developed breast cancer between 20 and 29 years of age

Fig. 5.5 Graphical risk explanation (remaining lifetime risk).

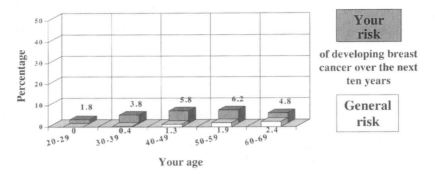

Fig. 5.6 Graphical risk explanation (10 yearly risk).

particular family history in comparison with remaining lifetime risk for general population (Fig. 5.5). This graph re-iterates the fact that as women grow older without developing cancer, they outlive some of their risk. In addition, the extra risk conferred by a family history decreases with age. The second graph shows 10 yearly absolute risks for a particular family history compared with population risks for different age groups (Fig. 5.6). A randomised controlled trial is underway to assess the effect of our method of risk explanation on risk perception and objective anxiety scores.

MANAGEMENT

In spite of extensive developments in molecular biology and genetics, it is not known how best to manage women who are at increased risk of developing breast cancer. The UK Family Cancer Study Group has recently published consensus guidelines to help clarify eligibility for genetic testing.[18]

SCREENING

Different clinics have different screening protocols and women as young as 25 years are able to get screening mammograms in the private sector. Though the value of mammography as a screening tool is not established in the under 50-year-olds, most family history clinics start screening mammography at 35 years for women at high- and moderate-risk. Though annual mammography may be justified in high-risk women, it is difficult to justify such intensive screening in the moderate-risk population especially at the lower end of the moderate-risk spectrum. Moreover, in light of recent findings of increased radiation sensitivity being associated with genetic predisposition to cancer,[19,20] annual mammography even in the high-risk group may do more harm than good. With the value of screening mammography in over 50-year-olds also under scrutiny, the time is ripe to have a randomised controlled trial of screening mammography in high-risk women. Other imaging modalities are also being looked at, and a multicentre trial is underway to define the role of magnetic resonance imaging in breast screening.

Key point 8–10

- Optimum management of women with a family history of breast cancer is under debate.

- Participation in chemopreventative and screening trials should be actively encouraged.

- The time is ripe for a randomised, controlled trial of screening mammography in moderate- and high-risk women.

CHEMOPREVENTION

Preventative drugs are also an issue. Tamoxifen has been licensed for use in the US following the results of the NSABP trial[21] that suggests that tamoxifen may decrease the incidence of breast cancer, although its efficacy in those with a genetic predisposition to the disease is far from clear. However, the long-term effects of tamoxifen were not evaluated because of the early closure of the trial and the efficacy of tamoxifen is still under trial in the UK, Australia and Europe (The International Breast Intervention Study).

Phytoestrogens are naturally occurring plant oestrogens. By virtue of their being ubiquitous in the Far-Eastern diet, where the incidence of breast cancer is low, they have been hypothesised to reduce breast cancer risk. However, their efficacy in reducing breast cancer risk has not been scientifically proven,[22] though they are freely available in health shops. We are currently performing a randomised controlled trial comparing the effect of two different doses of phytoestrogens and placebo on blood and urinary hormone levels and breast epithelial cell proliferation.

TRIALS

There is still much that is unknown about epidemiology, prevention, screening and management of women with an increased familial/genetic risk of breast cancer. Family history clinics, hence, have to be research-based and participation in clinical trials should be encouraged. However, in spite of the high level of motivation of these women, uptake into clinical trials is quite low. Part of the problem may be the differing views on risk assessment, screening and management offered by different clinics, especially if these women are seen in the symptomatic breast clinics. Uniformity of protocols should be an important contribution of stand-alone family history clinics. Recruitment of women into multicentre trials and prospective data collection should ultimately yield valuable information.

Key points for clinical practice

- Though genetic/familial cases contribute to only 5–10% of breast cancer cases, a close study of cancer families may add valuable information on gene–environment actions.

Key points for clinical practice *(continued)*

- Until a programme of risk assessment, screening and preventative management can be demonstrated to have a favourable effect on breast cancer mortality, family history clinics need to be research-based.

- Staff training, links with symptomatic, screening and genetic services and long-term funding should all be considered well in advance of starting a family history clinic.

- The family history clinic's referral criteria and management protocols should be consistent and widely circulated to general practitioners and other referrers to avoid inappropriate referrals.

- Risk assessment involves collection of family history data, drawing out a pedigree, ascertaining that breast and ovarian cancer are the predominant cancers and stratifying the family into a high-, moderate- or low-risk category.

- Numerical risk assessment can be done using the Gail, Claus or BRCAPRO models and their modifications.

- Women with a family history generally tend to overestimate their own risk of developing breast cancer. Even one-to-one risk counselling does not seem to have a long-term effect on an individual's personal risk perception.

- Optimum management of women with a family history of breast cancer is under debate.

- Participation in chemopreventative and screening trials should be actively encouraged.

- The time is ripe for a randomised, controlled trial of screening mammography in moderate- and high-risk women.

References

1. Eeles RA, Stratton MR, Goldgar DE, Easton DF. The genetics of familial breast cancer and their practical implications. Eur J Cancer 1994; 30A: 1383–1390.
2. Saunders C, Vijay V, Stein J, Baum M. Setting up a breast cancer family history clinic. Ann R Coll Surg Engl 1999; 81: 393–398.
3. Miki Y, Swensen J, Shattuck-Eidens D et al. A strong candidate for the breast and ovarian cancer susceptibility gene BRCA1. Science 1994; 266: 66–71.
4. Wooster R, Bignell G, Lancaster J et al. Identification of the breast cancer susceptibility gene BRCA2 [published erratum appears in Nature 1996; 379: 749]. Nature 1995; 378: 789–792.
5. Black WC, Nease Jr RF, Tosteson AN. Perceptions of breast cancer risk and screening effectiveness in women younger than 50 years of age [see comments]. J Natl Cancer Inst 1995; 87: 720–731.
6. Byrne GJ, Bundred NJ. Does the evidence justify national funding of breast cancer family history clinics? Breast 1997; 1997: 388–393.
7. Gail MH, Brinton LA, Byar DP et al. Projecting individualized probabilities of developing breast cancer for white females who are being examined annually [see comments]. J Natl Cancer Inst 1989; 81: 1879–1886.
8. Costantino JP, Gail MH, Pee D et al. Validation studies for models projecting the risk of invasive and total breast cancer incidence. J Natl Cancer Inst 1999; 91: 1541–1548.

9. Claus EB, Risch N, Thompson WD. Genetic analysis of breast cancer in the cancer and steroid hormone study. Am J Hum Genet 1991; 48: 232–242.

10. Claus EB, Risch N, Thompson WD. Autosomal dominant inheritance of early-onset breast cancer. Implications for risk prediction. Cancer 1994; 73: 643–651.

11. Parmigiani G, Berry D, Aguilar O. Determining carrier probabilities for breast cancer-susceptibility genes BRCA1 and BRCA2. Am J Hum Genet 1998; 62: 145–158.

12. Thirlaway K, Fallowfield L. The psychological consequences of being at risk of developing breast cancer. Eur J Cancer Prev 1993; 2: 467–471.

13. Smith BL, Gadd MA, Lawler C et al. Perception of breast cancer risk among women in breast center and primary care settings: correlation with age and family history of breast cancer. Surgery 1996; 120: 297–303.

14. Evans DG, Blair V, Greenhalgh R, Hopwood P, Howell A. The impact of genetic counselling on risk perception in women with a family history of breast cancer. Br J Cancer 1994; 70: 934–938.

15. Pharoah PDP, Mackay J. Absolute risk of breast cancer in women at increased risk: a more useful clinical measure than relative risk? Breast 1998; 1998: 255–259.

16. Cull A, Miller H, Porterfield T et al. The use of videotaped information in cancer genetic counselling: a randomized evaluation study. Br J Cancer 1998; 77: 830–837.

17. Lerman C, Lustbader E, Rimer B et al. Effects of individualized breast cancer risk counseling: a randomized trial. J Natl Cancer Inst 1995; 87: 286–292.

18. Eccles DM, Evans DG, Mackay J. Guidelines for a genetic risk based approach to advising women with a family history of breast cancer. J Med Genet 2000; 37: 203–209.

19. Angele S, Hall J. The ATM gene and breast cancer: is it really a risk factor? Mutat Res 2000; 462: 167–178.

20. Sharan SK, Morimatsu M, Albrecht U et al. Embryonic lethality and radiation hypersensitivity mediated by Rad51 in mice lacking BRCA2 [see comments]. Nature 1997; 386: 804–810.

21. Fisher B, Costantino JP, Wickerham DL et al. Tamoxifen for prevention of breast cancer: report of the National Surgical Adjuvant Breast and Bowel Project P-1 Study [see comments]. J Natl Cancer Inst 1998; 90: 1371–1388.

22. Ginsburg J, Prelevic GM. Lack of significant hormonal effects and controlled trials of phyto-oestrogens. Lancet 2000; 355: 163–164.

C.P. Shearman   Simon Boyes

CHAPTER 6

Carotid endarterectomy

Carotid endarterectomy (CEA) has been one of the most studied, yet controversial, surgical procedures of the last two decades. In 1905, Chiari first suggested emboli from the carotid artery might be a cause of stroke, a suggestion supported by the findings of Fisher who in 1950 demonstrated at post-mortem that the majority of fatal strokes were due to cerebral infarction associated with thrombo-embolic arterial disease. He also found that many of the subjects had atherosclerosis of the proximal, extracranial, internal carotid artery (ICA). The disease rarely extended much further than 1 cm from the carotid artery bifurcation prompting the suggestion that this might be surgically treatable.[1]

It was only one year later, in 1951, that this challenge was successfully taken up by a surgical team in Argentina operating on a patient with a progressive stroke. The diseased segment of ICA was resected and the healthy distal ICA anastomosed to the external carotid artery to restore cerebral circulation. DeBakey developed carotid thromboendartectomy in 1953 and Eastcote and his colleagues at St Mary's Hospital, London carried out a successful carotid resection in 1954 in a 66-year-old woman, which gained world-wide publicity.[2]

Due to its perceived role in stroke prevention, the number of carotid endarterectomies carried out in the US rapidly increased from 15,000 in 1971 to 107,000 in 1985.[3] However, concern regarding the role of CEA escalated, fuelled by the lack of consensus regarding the indications for intervention, the relatively poor results of surgery compared with medical treatment in some studies and the cost to the health care system.[4,5]

Prof. C.P. Shearman BSc MBBS MS FRCS, Head, Department of Vascular Surgery, E Level West Wing, Mail Point 67, Southampton General Hospital, Southampton SO16 6YD, UK (for correspondence)
Mr Simon Boyes BM FRCS, Vascular Research Fellow, Department of Vascular Surgery, E Level West Wing, Southampton General Hospital, Southampton SO16 6YD, UK

EVIDENCE FOR THE ROLE OF CEA

SYMPTOMATIC PATIENTS

The above concerns prompted a number of randomised controlled studies, two of which have made a major impact on the practice of carotid surgery. The European Carotid Surgery Trial (ECST) and the North American Symptomatic Carotid Endarterectomy Trial (NASCET) included patients with carotid artery disease who had had a non-disabling carotid artery territory stroke, transient ischaemic attack or retinal infarction (amaurosis fugax) within the previous 6 months. Patients were randomised to CEA plus best medical treatment or best medical treatment alone which entailed antiplatelet therapy (usually aspirin) and anti-hypertensive and anti-hyperlipidaemic drugs if indicated. Patients were grouped according to the measured severity of the carotid artery disease. In ECST, three groups were identified with mild (0–29%) moderate (30–69%) or severe (70–99%) ICA stenosis whereas NASCET randomised only those with severe (70–99%) and moderate (30–69%) disease. Unfortunately, the methods of estimating the degree of stenosis were different in the two studies, the ECST method producing a more severe stenosis when compared to NASCET method.

Interim reports of both studies appeared in 1991 and showed a clear benefit for surgery in patients with severe carotid artery disease and no benefit in those with mild disease. The final results of ESCT were published in 1998.[6] A total of 3024 patients were randomised with a mean follow-up of 6.1 years. The maximum benefit of surgery was apparent in patients with > 80% ICA stenosis when the risk of stroke or death at 3 years was 26.5% in the control group compared to 14.9% in those treated surgically, an absolute risk reduction of 11.6%. In order to prevent 1 stroke, 6 patients have to be submitted to CEA. Women suffered a higher complication rate from surgery suggesting the indication for them should be 90% ICA stenosis to gain optimum benefit. The stroke rate was highest in the first year in the medically treated group suggesting that surgery needed to be undertaken early after the neurological event to gain the maximum benefit. Long term results of NASCET demonstrated similar benefit from CEA in patients with severe stenosis of the ICA. At 8 years, the incidence of ipsilateral stroke was 14% after surgery compared to 27% in the medically treated group.[7] In patients with moderate stenosis, no benefit from surgery could be shown overall, but sub-group analysis in NASCET suggested a marginal benefit for patients with the more severe disease, 59–69% (equivalent to 70–80% in ECST). In practical terms, this means that 15 patients would have to be submitted to surgery to prevent 1 stroke in 5 years, which is probably unacceptable in most units. In both studies there was an associated stroke and death rate with surgery of 7.5% in ECST and 5.8% in NASCET. Patient selection criteria in the two studies were different, possibly explaining the difference between the trials, but these figures illustrate the need to keep complication rates to a minimum if CEA is to be of benefit.

ASYMPTOMATIC PATIENTS

Many patients with carotid artery atheroma have no related symptoms. These individuals appear to be at increased risk of stroke, but it is unclear whether CEA can reduce this risk. The prevalence of carotid disease rises from < 5% in those under 60 years of age to 10% in those over 80 years.[8] Although the cause of stroke is multifactorial, there does appear to be a relationship with carotid artery disease. Some 1820 patients with asymptomatic carotid disease showed an increase risk of stroke with increasing ICA stenosis. In the 60–90% stenosis group, the 5-year risk was 16.2% (3.2% annually). However, only 55% (1.9% annual risk) were thought to be caused by extracranial atheroma, the rest were related to intracranial disease or cardio-embolic causes.[9]

The Asymptomatic Carotid Atherosclerosis Study (ACAS), an American trial, showed a benefit in those patients undergoing CEA with a > 60% stenosis compared to the medically treated group. The estimated 5-year risk of ipsilateral stroke or any stroke or death was 11% in the medical group and 5.1% in the surgical group.[10] Several smaller studies have shown comparable marginal benefit. A meta-analysis of five of these trials, including ACAS, showed over an average duration of 3.1 years that the adjusted rate of ipsilateral stroke or any stroke or death in the medical group was 6.4% compared with 4.4% in those who had undergone CEA.[11] These results suggest that approximately 50 patients would require CEA to prevent one stroke over 3 years. ACAS has been criticised on a number of points as it was highly selective for both patient selection and centre inclusion. However, despite these concerns, the numbers of CEAs has risen from 46,571 in 1989 to 108,275 in 1996 when half of the procedures were for asymptomatic disease.[12] The large European based asymptomatic carotid trial (ACST) which includes 255 collaborators in 32 countries world-wide is still continuing and may reflect everyday practice more closely. Nearly 2500 patients with ICA stenosis 60–99% who have had no symptoms within the last 6 months have been randomised with a recruitment target of 3200 patients. It is hoped that this study will give some clear indications about the role of CEA in asymptomatic disease.[13,14]

OTHER INDICATIONS FOR CEA

Patients undergoing coronary artery bypass grafting (CABG) have a stroke risk of approximately 1%.[15] This is due to a number of factors including embolisation of atheroma from the aortic arch and problems associated with extra-corporal bypass. Significant ICA disease, however, is the strongest predictor of the risk of stroke and stroke rates in patients undergoing CEA in conjunction with CABG within the range for asymptomatic patients have been reported.[16] There is no evidence, however, that this approach reduces the stroke risk or is cost-effective. Most cardiac units have their own indications for combined CEA and CABG and, in our unit, we offer synchronous surgery to those patients with critical coronary artery disease and severe (70%) symptomatic carotid artery disease.

Some patients with extensive extracranial vascular disease with global symptoms thought to be due to cerebral hypoperfusion are offered CEA. The diagnosis is difficult to make and although reduced cerebral blood flow on isotope scan or loss of cerebrovascular reserve (the ability of the cerebral circulation to vasodilate during carbon dioxide inhalation) is supportive, there is no evidence that CEA will improve the situation.

Some patients will present with an evolving stroke thought to be due to carotid artery disease. It is generally held that intervention in such patients carries a very high risk of death. A few small studies have suggested that there may be benefit in urgent CEA in these situations, but the risks are high and the numbers of situations when this approach will be needed small, it seem sensible to confine this indication to units with a major interest in this field and when patients can be entered into trials.

INVESTIGATION OF PATIENT WITH SUSPECTED CAROTID ARTERY DISEASE

Before embarking on investigation, it is vital to establish that the patient has neurological symptoms compatible with emboli from the ICA. In practice this means a transient or permanent neurological deficit in the middle cerebral artery territory such as unilateral limb weakness, hemisensory loss, dysarthria or dysphasia or monoccular visual loss (amaurosis fugax) due to retinal artery occlusion. Global symptoms such as confusion, memory loss or bilateral symptoms are not generally associated with carotid artery disease. Ideally this process should be undertaken in close conjunction with a neurologist. It is also important to consider whether the patient would be fit for surgery if indicated and has neurological function worth preserving. A patient with a dense, non-resolving hemiparesis will gain little benefit from surgery.

The first line investigation for a patient with suspected carotid artery disease is duplex ultrasound scanning when both visualisation of the disease and determination of the degree of stenosis using Doppler can be achieved (Fig. 6.1). The direction of blood flow can be colour coded which aids the operator and speeds up the investigation. Colour flow duplex (CFD) has been shown to correlate well with arteriography in determining a degree of stenosis > 50%.[17,18] The non-invasive nature, lower cost and the accuracy of CFD means that it is the only specific investigation needed prior to surgery in the majority of patients. Problems arise in the presence of heavily calcified vessels where

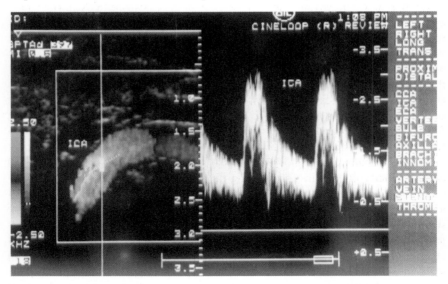

Fig. 6.1 Colour flow duplex scan of severe stenosis in internal carotid artery (ICA). B mode picture on left with Doppler waveform on right indicating blood flow velocity from which stenosis is estimated.

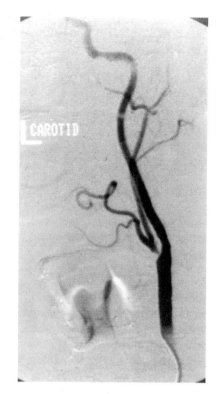

Fig. 6.2 Conventional angiogram showing stenosis at the origin of internal carotid artery.

CFD is significantly less reliable and it can be difficult to differentiate between severe stenosis and occlusion. This is a vital distinction as CEA is dangerous and of no benefit in the presence of complete ICA occlusion. Furthermore, CFD is unable to demonstrate the intracranial portion of the ICA and is also operator-dependent so that regular quality control measures need to be in place in any unit using it.

The gold standard for carotid artery imaging has been contrast arteriography that can give clear pictures of the disease and in particular identifies distal ICA disease (Fig. 6.2). However, there is an associated incidence of neurological complications between 0.5% and 4%[19] and in ACAS, 1.2% of patients had a cerebral infarct with arteriography.[10] The use of intra-arterial digital subtraction angiography may have gone some way to reducing this risk, although this has not been quantified.

Magnetic resonance angiography (MRA) demonstrated a sensitivity of 94% and specificity of 85% in determining carotid artery stenosis of 70–99%. The technology is fast improving, but not all equipment will produce such results and three-dimensional time of Flight (3D-TOF) produces an improvement in specificity.[20] MRA has a decreased sensitivity in assessing the intracranial ICA and is a poor predictor of ulceration of the atheromatous plaque. There is also concern about the ability of MRA to determine the difference between severe stenosis and occlusion, but improved scanning techniques and contrast agents such as gadolinium may overcome this problem.[21] Early reports of helical computed tomographic angiography (CTA) have proved promising. It uses a small volume of intravenous contrast and a short scan time of 30–40 s. Image

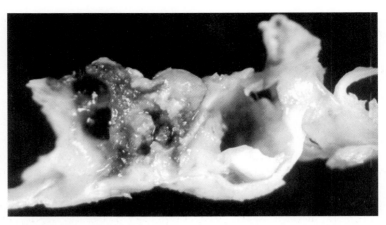

Fig. 6.3 Heterogeneous atheromatous plaque removed from internal carotid artery at endarterectomy in a symptomatic patient. Areas of haemorrhage, ulceration and platelet adherence can be seen.

acquisition is independent of flow and thus may be more accurate in identifying severe stenosis or occlusion. In addition, CTA may also give some indication of plaque morphology.[22,23]

The use of MRA and CFD can improve diagnostic accuracy to 94% with no false negatives.[12] There is still an indication for arteriography; however, in patients with suspected ICA occlusion or heavy calcified vessels where non-invasive imaging results do not correlate and when Duplex scanning has been technically difficult and the operator is not confident of the result.

PLAQUE MORPHOLOGY

Although degree of ICA stenosis is currently the strongest predictor of the risk of stroke and hence of the need for surgery in patients with carotid artery disease it is not the only factor. Atheroma is not a slowly progressive disease, but can undergo periods of intense cellular and inflammatory activity resulting in plaque haemorrhage or rupture (Fig. 6.3). These acute changes can result in distal embolisation or vessel occlusion and are related to clinical events such as myocardial infarction and stroke.[24] The presence of plaque ulceration correlates closely with the initial presentation of symptomatic patients.[25] This observation is supported by ECST data showing that plaque surface irregularity on angiography is associated with an increased ipsilateral stroke risk in patients with all degrees of stenosis risk even after years in those patients randomised to medical treatment.[26] The incidence of plaque haemorrhage is higher in those patients with a higher-grade stenosis.[23] The significance of this finding is unclear, but it has been suggested that the presence of haemorrhage promotes the development of atherosclerotic plaques.[27]

At the current time, the presence of plaque ulceration seems to have an influence on stroke rate. Apart from potentially identifying patients who may benefit from CEA, this observation also emphasises the important role of medical treatment. The benefit of antiplatelet agents such as low dose (75 mg) aspirin is clearly established,[28] but there is also interest in drugs such as statins, which may have a plaque stabilisation above and beyond their lipid lowering properties.[29]

TECHNICAL ASPECTS OF CEA

ANAESTHETIC

If the reported 30-day stroke and death rates of 5–10% could be reduced, this would add greater benefit to surgery. As complications of ischaemic heart disease are the commonest cause of death and most patients have wide-spread atherosclerotic vascular disease careful cardiovascular assessment is essential.[30]

A proportion of intra-operative neurological events are secondary to reduced cerebral blood flow at cross clamping and a lot of attention has been directed to preventing this (ironically the majority of peri-operative strokes are probably embolic).[31] Several methods have been used determine cerebral blood flow during surgery under general anaesthesia (GA) including transcranial Doppler ultrasound, electroencephalography and stump pressure. None of these have proved entirely reliable so some surgeons routinely use a shunt to maintain cerebral blood flow. The use of a shunt in those patients with decreased cerebral blood flow helps minimise the risk of ischaemic neurological events, but is associated with a risk of arterial dissection and embolic stroke.

It is suggested that a better assessment of neurological status can be made with the patient awake during the procedure using a superficial and deep cervical local anaesthetic block (LA). This allows early changes to be detected, particularly during cross clamping, and allows for the selective use of shunting. It also claimed that cerebrovascular autoregulation is preserved, unlike general anaesthetic (GA), allowing the patient to correct any small fluctuations in cerebral blood flow. A meta-analysis of 17 non-randomised and 3 randomised trials comparing GA with LA showed that LA might be beneficial in the reduction of early stroke, myocardial infarction and pulmonary complications. The use of shunting was also reduced in the LA group.[32] An additional benefit may be the lower cost of LA with shorter hospital stay and decreased use of intensive care. The piloting of the randomised controlled trial of GA versus LA (GALA) should objectively identify and advantages of LA. However it is unlikely that all patients will find LA CEA an acceptable procedure and surgeons who use vein to patch the artery find LA less acceptable.

SURGICAL

A linear arteriotomy along the ICA extending into the common carotid artery (CCA) is the commonest method of performing endarterectomy (Fig. 6.4). After endarterectomy, closure of the arteriotomy may be primary or with a patch using either autologous vein (Fig. 6.5) or prosthetic materials such as dacron or polytetrafluoroethylene (PTFE). A meta-analysis of six randomised trial and a more recent randomised trial of 399 patients has suggested that the use of a patch may confer a small reduction in peri-operative stroke rate. There

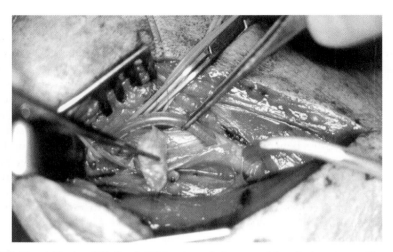

Fig. 6.4 Shunt (Burbank™, Bard, US) in place during carotid endarterectomy. The atheromatous plaque is being removed leaving a smooth medial surface. Reproduced with permission from Shearman.[41]

was also a significant reduction in the development of acute occlusion or long-term re-stenosis using a patch.[33,34] Currently no convincing evidence exists to recommend one patch material over another.[34,35] Vein is associated with a small risk of avascular necrosis and subsequent rupture which can be fatal. While the use of synthetic materials will preserve the saphenous vein and reduce the morbidity associated with harvesting it carries a higher risk of bleeding complications and infection.

Carotid eversion endarterectomy (CEE) was introduced in the early 1970s but only recently has it achieved much popularity.[36] The technique involves the division of the ICA at the bifurcation and an arteriotomy into the CCA. Once the plane of dissection is defined, the ICA is everted thus allowing the intima to strip away, resulting in easier completion of the endarterectomy. The endarterectomy of the common carotid is performed in the conventional

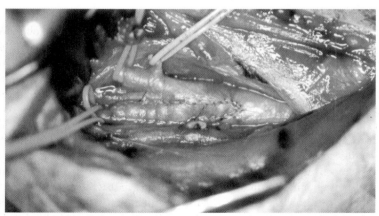

Fig. 6.5 Conventional carotid endarterectomy closed with patch of long saphenous vein. Reproduced with permission from Shearman.[41]

manner. The ICA is then re-implanted, with oblique excision of any redundant artery, onto the distal CCA. A prospective, randomised study comparing conventional CEA and PTFE patching with CEE in 336 endarterectomies in 310 patients showed some benefit in reducing peri-operative stroke (2.9% versus 0%) and death (0% versus 1.9%). There was also a reduction in clamping time (9 min versus 21 min) and the incidence of recurrent stenosis and late occlusive events were reduced.[37] Other retrospective studies have shown similar marginal benefits with CEE in reducing peri-operative stroke/death and occurrence of re-stenosis.

On completion of surgery, some form of quality check should be undertaken to identify technical errors such as intimal flaps which can be corrected. Completion angiography, TCD, Duplex or continuous wave ultrasound and angioscopy all have their advocates. The method chosen usually depends on local experience.

ENDOVASCULAR

The mortality and morbidity associated with CEA has prompted endovascular treatments of carotid artery disease. Despite concerns that angioplasty with or without stenting would result in embolisation and an unacceptable stroke rate, initial experience in a few centres suggested that the risks were low.[38] A number of series with very low stroke rates were published, but only 2 randomised studies have been reported. The Carotid and Vertebral Artery Transluminal Angioplasty Study (CAVATAS) reported all stroke and death rates in patients randomised to CEA or CA of 9.9% and 10%, respectively.[39] This study was criticised for the apparently poor surgical results compared to other series although the disabling stroke and death rate was 5.9% and 6.4%. A similar study was abandoned due to a high stroke rate in the angioplasty group.[40] A number of developments in stents and devices to prevent distal embolisation are being made. These together with better understanding of the plaque morphology may allow selection of patients suitable for CA with an added appeal of no risk of cranial nerve injury and reduced hospital stay.

SUMMARY

There is good evidence for the benefit of CEA symptomatic patients with a 80% stenosis of their ICA. The clinical and economic margins of benefit are very close and any unit undertaking this surgery needs to continually audit its results to ensure they remain acceptable with a death and stroke rate not more than 6%.[9] The benefit of CEA in asymptomatic patients is not clearly established, but ACST may provide clear answers. Available evidence would suggest that if surgery offers any advantage the margins of benefit would be extremely small and not very cost-effective as a method of stroke prevention. Improved visualisation of the plaque and identification of the highest risk group of patients may lead to optimum selection for surgery and identification of those patients more suitable for endovascular treatment Perhaps the brightest light on the horizon is not surgical but medical. Drugs that prevent rupture and induce stabilisation of the plaque may prevent the need for surgery in some patients.

Key points for clinical practice

- Symptomatic patients with >80% stenosis of ICA benefit from surgery

- Role of CEA in asymptomatic patients is unclear. Any beneffit is small

- The majority of patients can be treated on the results of Duplex ultrasound alone

- Local anaesthetic may have benefits for CEA and is being investigated in the GALA study

- The morphology of the atheromatous plaque appears to have prognostic significance.

References

1. Friedman SG. (ed) A History of Vascular Surgery. New York: Futura, 1989.
2. Eastcott HHG, Pickering GW, Rob CG. Reconstruction of internal carotid artery in a patient with intermittent attacks of hemiplegia. Lancet 1954; 267: 994–996
3. Pokras R, Dyken M. Dramatic changes in the performance of endarterectomy for disease of the extracranial arteries of the head. Stroke 1988; 19: 1289–1290.
4. Warlow C. Carotid endarterectomy: does it work? Stroke 1984; 15: 1068–1076.
5. Easton JD, Sherman DG. Stroke and mortality in carotid endarterectomy: 228 consecutive operations. Stroke 1977; 8: 565–568.
6. European Carotid Surgery Trialists' Collaborative Group. Randomised trial of endarterectomy for recently symptomatic carotid stenosis: final results of the MRC European Carotid Surgery Trial. Lancet 1998; 351: 1379–1387.
7. North American Symptomatic Carotid Endarterectomy Trial Collaborators. Benefit of carotid endarterectomy in patients with symptomatic moderate or severe disease. N Engl J Med 1998; 339: 1415–1425.
8. Prati P, Vanuzzo D, Casoroli M et al. Prevalence and determinants of carotid atherosclerosis in a general population. Stroke 1992; 23: 1705–1711.
9. Inzitari D, Eliasziw M, Gates P et al: The causes and risk of stroke in patients with asymptomatic internal carotid artery stenosis. N Engl J Med 2000; 342: 1693–1700.
10. Executive Committee for the Asymptomatic Carotid Atherosclerosis Study. Endarterectomy for asymptomatic carotid artery stenosis. JAMA 1995; 273: 1421–1428.
11. Benavente O, Moher D, Pham B. Carotid endarterectomy for asymptomatic carotid stenosis: a meta-analysis. BMJ 1998; 317: 1477–1480.
12. Karp HR, Flanders WD, Shipp CC, Taylor B, Martin D. Carotid endarterectomy among medicare beneficiaries: a state-wide evaluation of appropriateness and outcome. Stroke 1998; 29: 46–52.
13. Halliday AW, Thomas D, Mansfield A. The asymptomatic carotid surgery trial(ACST): rationale and design. Eur J Vasc Surg 1994; 8: 703–710.
14. Nicolaides AN. Asymptomatic carotid stenosis and risk of stroke: identification of a high risk group (ACSRS):a natural history study. Int Angiol 1995; 14: 21–23.
15. Renton S, Hornick P, Taylor KM, Grace PA. Rational approach to combined carotid and ischaemic heart disease. Br J Surg 1997; 84: 1503–1510.

16. Darling III RC, Dylewski M, Chang BB et al. Combined carotid endarterectomy and coronary artery bypass grafting does not increase the risk of perioperative stroke. Cardiovasc Surg 1998; 6: 448–452.

17. Polak JF, Bajakian RL, O'Leary DH et al. Detection of internal carotid artery stenosis: comparison of MR angiography, color Doppler sonography, and arteriography. Radiology 1992; 182: 35–40.

18. Erdoes LS, Marek JM, Mills JL et al. The relative contributions of carotid duplex scanning, magnetic resonance angiography, and cerebral arteriography to clinical decision making: a prospective study in patients with carotid occlusive disease. J Vasc Surg 1996; 23: 950–956.

19. Hankey GJ, Warlow CP, Sellar RJ. Cerebral angiographic risk in mild cerebrovascular disease. Stroke 1990; 21: 209–222.

20. Patel MR, Kuntz KM, Klufas RA et al. Pre-operative assessment of carotid bifurcation. Stroke 1995; 26: 1753–1758.

21. Willig DS, Turski PA, Frayne R et al. Contrast-enhanced 3D MR DSA of the carotid bifurcation: preliminary study of comparison with unenhanced 2D and 3D time-of-flight MR angiography. Radiology 1998; 208: 447–451.

22. Sameshima T, Futami S, Morita Y et al. Clinical usefulness of and problems with three-dimensional CT angiography for the evaluation of arteriosclerotic stenosis of the carotid artery: comparison with conventional angiography, MRA and ultrasound sonography. Surg Neurol 1999; 51: 300–309.

23. Cinat ME, Pham H, Vo D, Gordon I, Wilson SE. Improved imaging of carotid artery bifurcation using helical computed tomographic angiography. Ann Vasc Surg 1999; 13: 178–183.

24. Libby P, Geng YJ, Aikawa M et al. Macrophages and atherosclerotic plaque stability. Curr Opin Lipidol 1996; 7: 330–335.

25. Park AE, McCarthy WJ, Pearce WH, Matsumura JS, Yao JST. Carotid plaque morphology correlates with presenting symptomatology. J Vasc Surg 1998; 27: 872–879.

26. Rothwell PM, Gibson R, Warlow CP, on behalf of the European Carotid Surgery Trialists Collaborative Group. Interrelation between plaque surface morphology and degree of stenosis on carotid angiograms and the risk of ischaemic stroke in patients with symptomatic carotid stenosis. Stroke 2000; 31: 615–621.

27. Persson AV, Robichaux WT, Silverman M. The natural history of carotid plaque development. Arch Surg 1983; 118: 1048–1052.

28. Taylor W, Baenett HJM, Haynes RB et al. Low-dose and high dose acetylsalicyclic acid for patients undergoing carotid endarterectomy: a randomised controlled trial. Lancet 1999; 353: 2179–2184.

29. Haq I, Yeo W, Jackson P, Ramsay L. The case for cholesterol reduction in peripheral vascular disease. Crit Ischaemia 1997; 7: 15–22.

30. Riles TS, Kopelman I, Imparato AM. Myocardial infarction following carotid endarterectomy: a review of 683 operations. Surgery 1979; 85: 249–252.

31. Riles TS, Imparato AM, Jacobowitz GR et al. The cause of perioperative stroke after carotid endarterectomy. J Vasc Surg 1994; 19: 206–216.

32. Tangkanakul C, Counsell C, Warlow C. Local versus general anaesthesia for carotid endarterectomy (Cochrane review). Cochrane Database Syst Rev 2000.

33. Aburahma AF, Robinson PA, Saiedy S, Khan JH, Boland JP. Prospective randomized trial of carotid endarterectomy with primary closure and patch angioplasty with saphenous vein, jugular vein and polytetrafluoroethylene: long-term follow up. J Vasc Surg 1998; 27: 222–234.

34. Counsell C, Salinas R, Warlow C, Naylor R. Patch angioplasty versus primary closure for carotid endarterectomy. Cochrane Database Syst Rev 2000.

35. Counsell C, Warlow C, Naylor R. Patches of different types for carotid patch angioplasty. Cochrane Database Syst Rev 2000.

36. Etheridge SN. A simple technique of carotid endarterectomy. Am J Surg 1970; 120: 275–278.

37. Ballotta E, Da Giau G, Saladini M, Abbruzzese E, Renon L, Toniato A. Carotid endarterectomy with patch closure versus carotid eversion endarterectomy and re-implantation: a prospective randomized study. Surgery 1999; 125: 271–279.

38. Brown MM. Balloon angioplasty for cerebrovascular disease. Neurol Res 1992; 14 (suppl): 159–163.

39. Brown MM for the CAVATAS investigators. Results of the Carotid and Vertebral Artery Transluminal Angioplasty Study (CAVATAS). Cerebrovasc Dis 1998; 8 (suppl 4): 21.

40. Naylor AR, Bolia A, Abbott RJ et al. Randomised trial of carotid endarterectomy versus carotid angioplasty: a stopped trial. J Vasc Surg 1998; 28: 326–334.

41. Shearman CP. Carotid artery surgery. Lumley JSP, Craven JL, eds. Surgery 1993; 11: 416–420.

Simon John Hollingsworth Stephen George Edward Barker

Gene therapy in peripheral vascular disease

Interventional cardiovascular procedures are increasing year on year in an attempt to counter the effects of rising incidences in ischaemic heart, cerebrovascular and peripheral vascular disease (PVD).[1–3] Concomitantly, and unfortunately, post-procedural failures will become more common overall with arterial bypass grafts, for example, occluding in 20–35% of cases within 2 years from implantation and in specialist areas such as renal access, sometimes >50% of grafts placed occluding within 6 months.[4–15] Salvage procedures may help, but can prompt even higher secondary failure rates.[16–18]

Clearly, there is a real need for more varied (and effective) treatment options that are not necessarily 'interventional', or 'mechanical'. Furthermore, as modern day practice advances and becomes increasingly more specialised, the trend must be to become less and less invasive.

Over the last 20 years, through the application of recombinant DNA technology, there has been an exponential growth in the understanding of the molecular basis of both disease-free and disease states and an increasing ability to manipulate and control these processes. With this growing understanding, the challenge has become the translation and application of this knowledge base to provide useful and successful treatment protocols. A clear and attractive possibility is the use of DNA itself for therapy and it might just be a 'molecular' treatment, or 'gene therapy', of this type that offers the next significant advance for the peripheral vascular surgeon.

Here, we outline the basic principles of 'molecular modification' and 'gene therapy' as applied to PVD today and discuss in brief, how this can be performed. Finally, we highlight some of the clinical trials performed to date and speculate on what may come in the near future.

Dr S.J. Hollingsworth BSc PhD MPS, Lecturer in Molecular Medicine, The Academic Vascular Unit, Department of Surgery, The Royal Free and University College London Medical School, The Middlesex Hospital, Mortimer Street, London W1N 8AA, UK (for correspondence)
Mr S.G.E. Barker BSc MBBS MS FRCS, Senior Lecturer in Surgery, The Academic Vascular Unit, Department of Surgery, The Royal Free and University College London Medical School, The Middlesex Hospital, Mortimer Street, London W1N 8AA, UK

> ## Key point 1
>
> - Using DNA as a therapeutic may offer an alternative and attractive, less interventional option for the treatment of ischaemic heart, cerebrovascular and PVD.

BASIC PRINCIPLES OF VASCULAR GENE THERAPY

Somatic cell gene therapy uses a species of nucleic acid, or gene, as the therapeutic agent. For any proposed 'molecular' treatment, we require: (i) a knowledge of the gene, or nucleic acid sequence, of interest; (ii) an intended 'target' population of cells (or tissue) to be manipulated; (iii) a method to deliver the nucleic acid 'therapeutic' successfully to the site required; and (iv) a means to transfer the therapeutic to become effective once there.

The identification and isolation of particular genes, or sequences of interest, has become almost routine and an ever increasing number of candidates known to have at least some importance within the vasculature have been isolated (for examples, see Table 7.2.). The target populations of cells for vascular disease are, clearly, the endothelium, smooth muscle cells (SMCs) and those cells located in the adventitial tissues surrounding them. Molecular modification of these cell populations can be effected in essentially two ways: (i) ex vivo – whereby tissue is first removed from the body, modified in vitro and then, re-introduced back into the host; or (ii) in vivo – whereby the molecular modification is carried out in situ. Blood vessels represent one of the easiest targets for gene therapy as they are easy to access in situ, using either minimally-invasive endoluminal techniques or at open surgery.

METHODS OF GENE DELIVERY

Currently, one of three methods can be used to deliver the gene to the target tissue (i.e. a blood vessel, or its surrounding tissues) for in situ modification (for examples of each see below).

DIRECT INJECTION

The gene is injected directly into the tissues; either part of the blood vessel wall itself or, more commonly, into the muscle layers surrounding the area to be targeted.

> ## Key point 2
>
> - Molecular treatment requires knowledge of the gene of interest, an intended target population of cells, a method to deliver the nucleic acid therapeutic to the site required and a means to transfer the therapeutic into the target cells to become effective.

ENDOLUMINAL CATHETER DELIVERY

Using a double-ballooned catheter (Boston Scientific, USA; see Fig. 7.1.). Here,
a gene transfer solution is introduced into the luminal space created between
two inflated balloons. After perhaps 10–20 min, to allow for gene transfer to
occur, the balloons are deflated and the catheter removed.

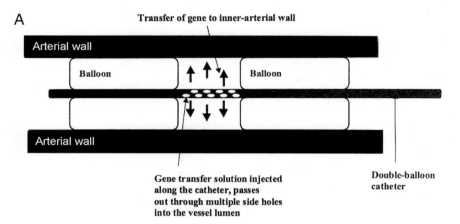

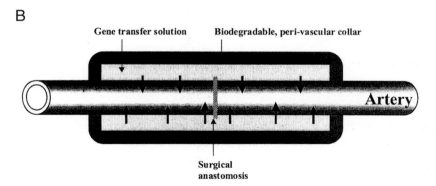

Fig. 7.1 Methods of arterial gene delivery. (**A**) Endoluminal. A double-balloon catheter
is passed endoluminally and the two (separate) balloons are inflated. Through a
central channel in the catheter, the gene transfer solution is injected into the lumen of
the vessel, through multiple side-holes in the catheter. After ~10–20 min (to allow
gene transfer) the balloons are deflated and the catheter withdrawn. (**B**) Peri-vascular.
When vessels are exposed at surgery, the vessel (particularly, around an anastomosis)
can be encased in a biodegradable, perivascular arterial collar, or capsule, which is
then sealed. The gene transfer solution is then injected directly into the space between
the inner capsule wall and the outer surface of the vessel. Gene transfer is via the
adventitial surface of the vessel.

PERIVASCULAR COLLAR DELIVERY

Used at the time of open surgery, when the blood vessels are directly exposed (see Fig. 7.1.). Here, a biodegradable, perivascular capsule, or collar (Eurogene Limited, UK), is placed and sealed around the outside of an artery and a gene transfer solution introduced into the space between them. Gene transfer is to the adventitial surface of the blood vessel.

Whichever method is used to deliver the gene to the specific site required, the gene of interest must then be transferred into the relevant cell population targeted, so as to become effective. However, if naked DNA alone is used and placed in contact with cell membranes, only an extremely small percentage will pass into the cells. Therefore, to increase the level of gene transfer, one of two gene transfer systems is often used.

- **Non-viral gene transfer** –where genes are encapsulated within, or associated with, a 'carrier molecule' such as a liposome.

- **Viral gene transfer** – whereby the gene is contained within a viral vector system that relies on the natural infectious properties of the virus employed, to transfer the gene.

The choice of whether to use non-viral or viral gene transfer will be determined by a number of factors which include principally; (i) the efficiency of transfer required to obtain the desired therapeutic effect; (ii) the size of the gene of interest that is to be transferred; (iii) the duration of gene expression required following transfer, (iv) whether the modification required is to be heritable (i.e. does the gene need to integrate into the host-cell genome); (v) whether, or not, the cells of the target tissue are dividing; (vi) whether the cells, once modified, will become a target susceptible to host immune attack; and (vii) whether there are any particular safety features to note, or limitations, with the method chosen.

NON-VIRAL GENE TRANSFER

For non-viral gene transfer any of the following methods may be employed:[19,20]

- **Direct injection** – as described above (this may be performed also under a microscope into single cells).

- **Calcium phosphate precipitation** – during which the cell membrane is rendered temporarily porous to allow the DNA through.

- **Electroporation** – whereby a small electric charge is applied across cells in suspension, rendering the cell membranes porous to the DNA.

- **Cationic lipids** – where DNA is complexed to, or contained within, lipid spheres, which on contact with cell membranes, fuse and introduce the DNA into the cell. In addition, attempts have been made to target lipids more efficiently by including within their structure, ligands to known target tissue receptors.

- **Particle bombardment/'gene gun'** – where DNA is coated on to the surface of small, gold or tungsten beads which are then 'fired' at cells using either an electric discharge, or gas pulse, with the physical force of impact overcoming the membrane barrier and hence, introducing the DNA into the cell.

- **Receptor-mediated gene transfer** – where the DNA might be complexed to a ligand of a known receptor on the target cell surface, using receptor-mediated internalisation to transfer the DNA.

Clearly, some of these methodologies are not suitable for in situ gene transfer and for vascular gene delivery it is most common to use direct, naked DNA injection, DNA/liposome complexes, or a combination of DNA complexed to receptor-mediated/targeted liposomes.

VIRAL GENE TRANSFER

Viruses were first considered as a vehicle ('vector') by which to transfer DNA due to their natural ability to infect cells within the human body and successfully transfer their own genome to the host cell, to enable viral propagation. With modifications, for obvious safety reasons, viruses can be employed as an efficient means to transfer ('infect') DNA into a cell. Although many different viruses are being investigated and developed for gene transfer,[20] by far the most commonly used are:

- **Retro-viruses**[20,21] – the most commonly used viral system due to our current level of understanding and experience, but whose major limiting feature is an inability to infect non-replicating cells.

- **Adeno-viruses**[20,22] – which achieve the highest levels of gene transfer of any of the viral systems employed to date and which can transfer DNA into either replicating, or non-replicating, cells.

Other viral systems currently being tested and developed (but yet to be applied clinically) include many of the Herpes viruses, adeno-associated viruses, Semliki Forest virus lenti-viruses, Sinbis viruses as well as 'kit' viruses (artificially fabricated from components of other viruses) and a whole host of other new 'viral-like' systems.[20–23]

Common to most viral gene transfer systems is the necessity to produce a virus that can infect the target cell/tissue once only ('single-step') and which can not subsequently, produce infectious virus able to go on and infect other ('non-target') cells and tissues. This can be achieved by producing a 'disabled virus', through the intermediate step of a 'packaging cell (line)'. To do this, a vector is constructed containing the gene(s) of choice, in combination with an essential controlling sequence from the virus genome (for example, in the case of retro-viruses, this is most often the packaging signal). In a separate gene construct, the virus genome is re-constructed containing those genes required for propagation, but excluding the essential controlling sequence. Both constructs are then transferred into the packaging cell. Here, within this cell, although the virus can produce all of the proteins and enzymes it requires for its normal life cycle, the essential controlling sequence allowing an infectious particle to be produced and packaged is missing – hence, a disabled virus. However, this controlling sequence is present in conjunction with the gene(s) of choice within the packaging cell and so, a 'single-step' infectious particle is produced, or packaged, that contains the gene of choice and not the virus

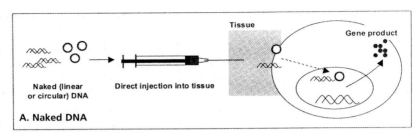

A. Naked DNA

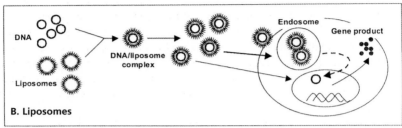

B. Liposomes

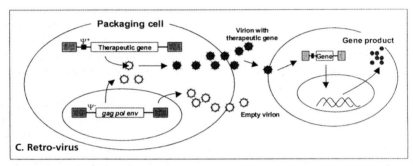

C. Retro-virus

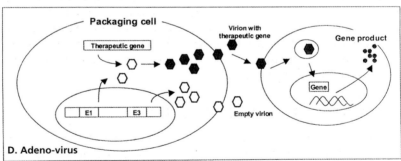

D. Adeno-virus

Fig. 7.2 Viral and non-viral methods of gene transfer.[19–23] **(A)** Naked DNA. Naked DNA is injected using a transfer solution (such as normal saline) into the tissues of the area required – this can be surrounding muscle tissue, or the vessel wall itself. DNA crosses the cell membrane on contact. **(B)** Liposomes. DNA is complexed to cationic lipids which, on contact with the cell membrane, aid in the transfer of DNA into the cell. **(C)** Retro-viruses. A packaging cell is produced containing the therapeutic gene in combination with an essential part of the virus genome (the packaging signal required to package the virus into an infective viral particle). The remaining genes of the viral genome are placed on separate DNA constructs within the cell. The packaged virions produced by the cell contain only the gene therapeutic. These infective viral particles (in a transfer solution) are then used to transfer the gene therapeutic into the target cell. **(D)** Adeno-viruses. As with retro-viruses, a packaging cell is created that produces infectious adeno-virus particles containing only the gene therapeutic. These infective viral particles (in solution) are then used to transfer the gene therapeutic into the target cell.

genome. These disabled viral particles can now be used to infect the target population of cells (Fig. 7.2).[20–22]

Although a detailed critique of the viral and non-viral methods of gene transfer is beyond the scope of this article, it can be found elsewhere.[19–23] However, in brief, non-viral gene transfer systems are the safest to use, but confer only a very low efficiency of gene transfer which often, can be the limiting factor in their use. In contrast, viral systems confer a far greater efficiency of gene transfer, but have associated safety issues such as retaining the possibility of producing infectious virus once transferred (due to homologous recombination, or a previous viral infection), or the potential (in some systems) for insertional mutagenesis.

In those clinical applications of vascular gene therapy tried to date, the most commonly used methods have been; for non-viral gene transfer – naked plasmid DNA and plasmid/liposome complexes, and for viral gene transfer – retro-viruses and adeno-viruses. Figure 7.2 demonstrates how these systems are used to transfer the gene of interest and Table 7.1 summarises the main characteristics, advantages and disadvantages of each.

No single gene transfer system is likely to be applicable to all areas of vascular gene therapy due to the varied nature of the underlying disease processes involved and the differing requirements for gene delivery, control and duration of expression. To this extent, new, mainly viral systems are being developed and tested. Undoubtedly, improvements in these technical areas will offer the greatest challenge to allow clinical gene therapy to be more widely applied in vascular (and other) diseases.

For most vascular disorders, however, a beneficial biological effect might be achieved with very low levels (<1%) of gene transfer and with only temporary expression of the genes, once transferred.[23–25] The requirements of the gene delivery system and control of the gene once transferred might, therefore, be less crucial than for example, in diseases such as cystic fibrosis, or cancer, where often long-term expression is required to maintain the desired therapeutic effect. Not only does this reduce some of the technological advances needed to make vascular gene therapy a more common place reality, but it may allow also, the use of gene transfer systems that offer increased safety over those systems that concentrate on improved gene transfer efficiency alone.

TARGETS FOR VASCULAR GENE THERAPY

Our increasing knowledge of the molecular regulation of the vasculature has led to the identification of a significant number of genes that appear as clear candidates for effecting a therapy. Table 7.2 summarizes a number that might be used as a 'therapeutic' in PVD. For example, if the underlying disease problem is

---

Key point 4

- The transfer of genes across the cell membrane to become effective in the target population of cells can be by non-viral methods that employ more physical means of transfer, or by viral gene transfer vectors that rely on the natural infectious properties of the viruses used.

Table 7.1 Main characteristics, advantages and disadvantages of gene transfer systems in current vascular gene therapy[19–23]

(A) Non-viral gene transfer. Advances in lipid formulae and synthetic cationic polymer carriers have improved the efficiency of plasmid/liposome-mediated gene transfer.[41–43] Additionally, attempts are being made to embed within the lipid layer, ligands to cell surface specific receptors, to enhance gene transfer by receptor-mediated processes.[38]

Transfer system – Naked plasmid DNA

Main characteristics	*Route of transfer*
Linear or circular DNA	Direct contact with cell membrane or injection into tissues
Advantages	*Disadvantages*
* Easy to produce	• Low efficiency of gene transfer
* Safety	• Transient gene expression
	• Difficult to obtain stable gene transfer

Transfer system – Plasmid DNA/liposomes

Main characteristics	*Route of transfer*
Linear or circular DNA complexed to/within liposomes	Direct contact with cell membrane
Advantages	*Disadvantages*
• Easy to produce	• Low efficiency of of gene transfer
• Safety	• Transient gene expression
• Efficiency>naked DNA alone	• Difficult to obtain stable gene transfer
• Can target liposomes to specific receptors	

Transfer system – Oligonucleotides

Main characteristics	*Route of transfer*
Linear, single-stranded DNA targeted against a known mRNA species	Direct contact with cell membrane
Advantages	*Disadvantages*
• Easy to produce	• Degradability
• Low cost	• A 'one hit' option
• Safety	

(B) Viral gene transfer. New, 'pseudo-typed' retro-viruses, with the virus capsid containing a protein to a known cell type specific receptor, have permitted both increased viral titres and more efficient gene transfer.[38]

Transfer system – Retro-virus

Main characteristics	*Route of transfer*
• Diploid, positive-strand RNA virus (9.2 kb)	Receptor-mediated
• Maximum gene insert of 8 kb	
• Location – nuclear	
Advantages	*Disadvantages*
• More efficient gene transfer	• Only effective in proliferating cells
• Stable integration	• Possibility of insertional mutagenesis
• Long-term, durable gene expression	• Potential for production of replication competent virus
• Clinical experience	• Complex to produce
	• Low viral titres (10^6–10^8 cfu/ml)
	• Needs packaging cell
	• Limited size for gene insert
	• Host immunological response
	• Loss of gene expression by LTR methylation

Transfer system – Adeno-virus

Main characteristics	*Route of transfer*
• Double-stranded, linear DNA virus (36 kb)	Receptor-mediated
• Maximum gene insert of ~8 kb	
• Location – nuclear	
Advantages	*Disadvantages*
• Effective in non-dividing and dividing cells	• Transient gene expression
• Effective transient gene expression	• Does not integrate
• Does not integrate	• Complex production
• High viral titres (10^8–10^{10} cfu/ml)	• Limited size for gene insert
	• Needs packaging cell
	• Host immunological and inflammatory response (has caused deaths in trials)
	• Safety issues

Table 7.2 Genes of interest by therapeutic target[23]

Therapeutic target	Potential mechanism(s)	Potential therapeutic genes/targets	
'Ischaemia'	Genes to stimulate new blood vessel growth – 'therapeutic angiogenesis' Genes to help vasodilatation	VEGF-A, -B, -C, -D, -E FGF-1, -2, -4, -5 Angiopoietin-1, -2 Hepatocyte growth factor	MCP-1 PDGF-BB eNOS, iNOS
Atherosclerosis	Reduce oxidative stress Increase oxygenation Reduce lipid uptake Modulate lipid modification/metabolism/oxidation	LDL receptor apoE, apoA-1, apoAI_Milano Lipoprotein lipase Hepatic lipase apoB editing enzyme Lipid transfer proteins	LCAT Lp(a) inhibition Soluble VCAM Soluble ICAM Anti-oxidative enzymes
SMC-NIH (promoting stenosis and re-stenosis)	Genes to prevent smooth muscle cell proliferation Genes to block proliferative signals Apoptosis-inducing genes Tumour-suppresser genes Genes involved in intracellular signalling or cycle regulation	VEGF-A, -C eNOS, iNOS TIMPs, COX tk, gax, CyA p53, Rb fas ligand p16, p21, p27	c-myb, c-myc cdk-2, cdc-2 NKkB and E2F decoys ras, bcl, Gβγ PCNA antisense Oligonucleotides Hammerhead ribozymes Blocking PDGF or TGF-β expression or receptors
Thrombosis	Reduce thrombogenicity Modulate thrombosis	tPA COX	Thrombomodulin Hirudin
Aneurysm formation	Modulate vessel wall re-modelling Prevent enzymatic degradation of vessel wall	TIMPs TGF-βb	

VEGF, vascular endothelial growth factor; FGF, fibroblast growth factor; MCP-1, monocyte chemotactic protein-1; PDGF, platelet-derived growth factor; NOS, nitric oxide synthase; TIMP, tissue inhibitor of metalloproteinase; COX, cyclo-oxygenase; tk, thymidine kinase; CyA, cytosine deaminase; Rb, retinoblastoma; PCNA, proliferating cell nuclear antigen; TGF-β, transforming growth factor beta; LDL, low-density lipoprotein; LCAT, lectin-cholesterol acyl-transferase; VCAM, vascular-cell adhesion molecule; ICAM, intercellular adhesion molecule; tPA, tissue plasminogen activator.

related to ischaemia, then it might be considered logical to use a therapeutic that stimulates the growth of new blood vessels, thereby increasing blood flow to the affected area – an approach known as 'therapeutic angiogenesis'. Alternatively, for example, in attempting to treat SMC-NIH, it would seem reasonable to deliver genes that might arrest SMC proliferation, either by a direct action, or through the blockade of a growth-stimulatory signal.

Key point 5

- Targets for gene therapy in PVD include stimulation of angiogenesis to help reduce ischaemia, controlling smooth muscle cell growth to help prevent stenosis and re-stenosis, and intervening in the atherosclerotic and thrombotic disease processes.

Depending on the specific disease target and the gene chosen as the therapeutic, it is likely that one of the following approaches will be employed.

Gene addition

Consists of either: (i) insertion into a cell of either a new gene to enable production of a protein not normally expressed by that cell type; or alternatively, (ii) an additional copy of a gene to enhance, or elevate, production of a particular protein that might normally be expressed by that cell type. For example, an additional copy of genes to elevate production of angiogenic proteins, such as vascular endothelial growth factor (VEGF), or basic fibroblast growth factor (bFGF), might be used to combat ischaemia. Alternatively, genes such as that for nitric oxide synthase, may aid in vessel dilatation and vascular tone regulation.

Control of gene expression

Whereby alteration of the control of a particular gene is effected by using nucleic acid sequences to target either those sequences in DNA used to control gene expression, or alternatively, to target specific species of RNA to prevent protein production.

Gene replacement

Consists of the substitution of a non-active, or defective gene by a new, or additional, functional copy of the gene to restore the production of a required protein.

Principally, in clinical trials performed to date, gene addition and control of gene expression have been used (see below).

Key point 6

- Effecting PVD gene therapy may involve gene replacement, gene addition or control of gene expression.

VASCULAR GENE THERAPY IN THE CLINIC

The translation of experimental gene therapy for PVD into the clinical setting is a relatively new event, apparent only within the last 5 years or so. Accordingly, most early studies have focused on safety testing, developing delivery systems and overall feasibility (phase I studies). Although in some studies, efficacy has been a secondary end-point, it is important to note that many (early) phase I safety studies were performed in patients with 'end-stage' disease who were (possibly) less likely to respond to treatment than those individuals for whom the treatment is ultimately targeted. The regulatory processes currently in force, require that safety testing can not be performed in patients for whom more traditional treatments are likely to have some efficacy already. It is, however, these very individuals who would probably be more likely to respond. That said, for the trials performed to date, although there are few published reports, early results have been encouraging and the efficacy with treatment seen in some cases clearly suggests a potential for this type of treatment to be more widely applied.

In 1995, Isner and co-workers performed one of the first gene therapy trials for cardiovascular disease, in non-diabetic patients with rest pain and ischaemic ulceration of the lower limbs.[26] The approach taken was to try and reduce ischaemia by stimulating angiogenesis, through the delivery of VEGF (therapeutic angiogenesis) to the affected tissues. Patients received escalating doses of VEGF-DNA, delivered to the luminal endothelium (of the profunda femoris artery) using an angioplasty balloon, precoated with a hydro-gel polymer containing a VEGF plasmid-DNA vector. The preliminary findings showed a promising clinical response as evidenced by an increase in peripheral blood flow and some alleviation of symptoms (in 3 of the 7 patients treated). Similarly, Baumgartner and colleagues (in 1998) adopted the approach of therapeutic angiogenesis and used VEGF plasmid-DNA in patients with ischaemic limbs, with non-healing ulcers and rest pain.[27] Here, DNA transfer was by direct injection into the leg muscles surrounding the ischaemic area. Significantly, the treatment prompted improved ankle-brachial pressure indices, with contrast angiography showing increased collateral blood vessel formation in 7 of 10 limbs. Furthermore, the ischaemic ulcers either healed, or improved substantially, in 4 of 7 limbs. Successful limb salvage proved possible in three patients who had been advised previously, to undergo below-knee amputation.

This approach of therapeutic angiogenesis has been the treatment most widely employed to date, on the assumption that for an ischaemic condition, the stimulation of new blood vessel growth to increase oxygen delivery to the tissues is likely to be most beneficial. Currently, intramuscular injection is being used in the treatment of PVD to deliver: (i) naked DNA for VEGF-A[27,28] or VEGF-C;[29] (ii) plasmid DNA (pCOR), containing fibroblast growth factor-1;[30] and (iii) adeno-virus vector, containing the gene for fibroblast growth factor-4.[31] Intramuscular injection of naked VEGF-A DNA is being used also for the treatment of Buerger's disease.[32] Furthermore, hydro-gel-coated, or infusion-perfusion balloon catheters are being employed for the treatment of PVD, or post-percutaneous transluminal angioplasty re-stenosis, to deliver: (i) liposome-complexed adeno-virus, containing the gene for VEGF-A;[33] and (ii) in preliminary safety and gene transfer studies, adeno-virus containing the marker gene *lac-Z*.[34]

More recently, the problem of SMC-NIH causing stenosis following arterial bypass grafting, or re-stenosis following angioplasty, has become a target for vascular gene therapy. If delivered (at the time of surgery, or angioplasty) to those sites where SMC proliferation causes most problems, genes that can modulate SMC function may have some potential in preventing SMC-NIH (see also Table 7.2). In attempting to treat SMC-NIH, the gene of choice may be delivered to the arterial wall either endoluminally or alternatively, from the outside, i.e. at the adventitial surface. If attempting to prevent re-stenosis following angioplasty, however, the obvious approach is to use another balloon catheter (double-balloon catheter, Boston Scientific, USA; see Fig. 7.1) as the gene may be transferred at the same time as the angioplasty is being performed. Currently, this approach is being used to deliver the gene for VEGF-A contained within an adeno-virus and complexed to liposomes.[33] Results from this trial should be available soon. In contrast, for the prevention of stenosis following arterial bypass grafting, although endoluminal gene delivery is possible (by means of a balloon catheter sometime following surgery) different approaches are being employed. A biodegradable, arterial collar, placed around the outside of the artery (at the sites of surgical anastomosis) and sealed at either end (Eurogene Limited, UK; see Fig. 7.1) enables the adventitial surface of the artery (and adjacent bypass conduit) to be bathed in a solution containing the gene of interest, together with an appropriate transfer agent. Experimental models have demonstrated this to be a feasible method[24,25] and currently, this is being employed to deliver a gene for VEGF contained within a plasmid vector and complexed to liposomes, aimed at minimising graft failure due to SMC-NIH following bypass.[35]

In an alternative strategy, the problem of arterial bypass graft failure has been approached using a method of ex vivo gene therapy.[36] Here, autologous veins from patients undergoing first time, or repeat, infra-inguinal arterial bypass grafting were harvested and then placed first, into a solution containing a decoy oligonucleotide designed to bind to, and inactivate, the pivotal cell-cycle transcription factor, E2F. The gene transfer solution was then pressurized for 10 min (without undue distention of the vein), to enable oligonucleotide transfer. The modified veins were then replaced as bypass grafts.

In sections of vein modified but not used as a bypass graft, a gene transfer efficiency of 89% was achieved. Notably, molecular markers of cellular proliferation (proliferating cell nuclear antigen and *c-myc* mRNA) were reduced significantly . Postoperative complication rates were unaffected by treatment but significantly, in comparison to patients receiving autologous vein grafts that were not modified, fewer graft occlusions, revisions, or critical stenoses were seen at 12 months following surgery.

In the only other reported example of ex vivo gene therapy for PVD, primary hepatocytes were transduced (using a retrovirus) to express the gene for low-density-lipoprotein (LDL), before re-introduction into patients with familial hypercholesterolaemia, the aim being to help reduce the risk of developing atherosclerosis.[37] Here, in 3 of the 5 patients treated, a significant and prolonged reduction was demonstrated in LDL cholesterol. Furthermore, in a previously LDL receptor-negative patient, in vivo LDL catabolism was increased by 53% and there was an associated significant reduction in their serum LDL.

Key point 7

- Early clinical trials have demonstrated gene therapy to be of potential benefit in the treatment of ischaemia (by stimulating angiogenesis), bypass graft failure (by inhibiting SMC proliferation), and atherosclerosis (by reducing serum LDL cholesterol and improving LDL cholesterol catabolism).

Results from many other trials currently being performed should be available within 2–3 years and probably, it will not be until the publication of these results that we truly begin to see the potential of gene therapy in PVD. So far, anecdotally, results seem promising.

CURRENT LIMITATIONS OF VASCULAR GENE THERAPY

The main issues limiting the application of vascular gene therapy clinically are in the delivery, and transfer, of genes to the tissues required and thence, control of the genes once transferred. Although the methods currently in use such as the peri-vascular arterial collar and double-balloon catheter allow a site-directed gene delivery, transfer of the gene is not confined to any particular cell type. The importance of this is not yet clear. However, it is reasonable to postulate that by enabling specific cell types to express particular genes, this may be of greater therapeutic benefit. For example, if SMCs only can be modified to express VEGF, then this should be preferable to having surrounding fibroblasts expressing VEGF also. The rationale behind this is several fold: (i) initially, this may be more in keeping with the normal physiology of the vessel wall; (ii) it is a normal function of SMCs to produce molecules such as VEGF, whilst this may not be the case for fibroblasts and accordingly, we do not know the consequences of cells now fashioning molecules that they would not normally produce; (iii) modification of cells to express molecules that would not normally be produced may alter overall cellular function, or in other circumstances, may stimulate an inappropriate host-immune response; or (iv) the transfer of genes to non-target cells may reduce overall transfer efficiency and effectiveness, either if the gene is rendered non-active, in non-target tissue (as production of the molecule is not a normal function of that cell type), or simply, by diluting the overall amount of gene transferred to the desired site. Clearly, a major area of interest for the future of gene therapy lies in the development of more accurate, and efficient, delivery and transfer systems.

Equally as important, however, is our ability to control the gene once transferred. Maintaining gene expression, or controlling expression, to a specific level (or even to 'high' or 'low' levels) is as yet, a major technical hurdle still to overcome. With the expected development of more sophisticated systems in this area far more effective 'molecular intervention' should become feasible.

> **Key point 8**
>
> - Improvements in gene transfer technology and our ability to control genes once transferred will help see gene therapy a more common-place reality for the treatment of PVD.

Despite these current limitations, however, targeting gene transfer to specific cell types by cell-specific receptor mechanisms, or controlling gene expression through the use of cell type-specific gene promotors, is being explored and becoming more and more a reality.[38–40]

PROSPECTS FOR VASCULAR GENE THERAPY

Our understanding of the molecular mechanisms underlying many of the disease processes dominant in PVD is, undoubtedly, at an early stage. Only when we have a much fuller and clearer understanding of these processes and so, more detailed information as to the levels of gene expression required, or the mechanisms by which to control the gene activation that is inherent, will we be in a more appropriate position to try and effect intervention.

Similarly, gene delivery and transfer systems are in their infancy. However, early ventures have demonstrated a clear potential for the application of gene therapy in the future. In the short-to-medium term, it is most likely that gene therapy will serve as an adjuvant to more conventional therapies, or as an experimental therapeutic alternative once these have been exhausted. However, as experience increases, combined with an enhanced knowledge of the molecular basis of disease as well as genetic screening programs, it may become possible to target individuals at risk, to intervene and to treat, or vaccinate, against the onset of disease prior to other, more radical, treatments being required.

In the near future, however, it may be possible and indeed sensible, to apply gene therapy to more common, less 'end-stage' problems such as the local treatment of venous and diabetic ulceration, whereby genetic manipulation of growth factors may assist in wound healing. Possibly, this might be combined with a simultaneous 'gene therapy' directed systemically to treat the underlying vascular, or diabetic, disease process.

In time, it may become possible to develop a 'time therapeutic', whereby individuals could be vaccinated early in life using a gene transfer system that locates itself to the specific site required, only to become activated when that specific disease process starts – somewhat akin to an anti-virus programme that runs on a computer.

> **Key points for clinical practice**
>
> - Using DNA as a therapeutic may offer an alternative and attractive, less interventional option for the treatment of ischaemic heart, cerebrovascular and PVD.

Key points for clinical practice (continued)

- Molecular treatment requires knowledge of the gene of interest, an intended target population of cells, a method to deliver the nucleic acid therapeutic to the site required and a means to transfer the therapeutic into the target cells to become effective.

- For the treatment of PVD, gene delivery to the site required can be by direct injection into the tissues, by endoluminal catheter, or by a perivascular collar.

- The transfer of genes across the cell membrane to become effective in the target population of cells can be by non-viral methods that employ more physical means of transfer, or by viral gene transfer vectors that rely on the natural infectious properties of the viruses used.

- Targets for gene therapy in PVD include stimulation of angiogenesis to help reduce ischaemia, controlling smooth muscle cell growth to help prevent stenosis and re-stenosis, and intervening in the atherosclerotic and thrombotic disease processes.

- Effecting PVD gene therapy may involve gene replacement, gene addition or control of gene expression.

- Early clinical trials have demonstrated gene therapy to be of potential benefit in the treatment of ischaemia (by stimulating angiogenesis), bypass graft failure (by inhibiting SMC proliferation), and atherosclerosis (by reducing serum LDL cholesterol and improving LDL cholesterol catabolism).

- Improvements in gene transfer technology and our ability to control genes once transferred will help see gene therapy a more common-place reality for the treatment of PVD.

References

1. European Working Group on Critical Leg Ischaemia. Second European Consensus Document on Chronic Critical Leg Ischaemia. Eur J Vasc Surg. 1992; 6 (Suppl A): 103–141.
2. Wolfe JHN, Harris PL, Vaughan Ruckley C. Trust hospitals and vascular services. BMJ 1994; 309: 414–419.
3. Hillegass WB, Ohman EM, Califf RM. Restenosis: the clinical issues. In: Topol EJ. (ed) Textbook of Interventional Cardiology. Philadelphia PA: 1994, 415–435.
4. Smith SH, Gear JC. Morphology of saphenous vein coronary artery bypass grafts. Arch Pathol Lab Med 1983; 107: 13–19.
5. **Bulkley BH, Hutchins GM. Accelerated 'athersclerosis'. A morphological study of 97 saphenous vein coronary artery bypass grafts. Circulation 1977; 55: 163–166.**
6. **Ratliff NB, Myles TH. Rapidly progressive 'atherosclerosis' in aortocoronary saphenous vein grafts. Arch Pathol Lab Med 1989; 113; 772–775.**
7. Mills JH, Taylor SM. Results of infra-inguinal revasculization with reversed vein conduits. Ann Vasc Surg 1991; 5: 156–160.
8. Mills JH, Fujitami RM, Taylor SM. The characteristics and anatomic distribution of lesions that cause reversed vein graft failure. J Vasc Surg 1993; 17: 195–197.
9. Bandyk DF, Mills TH. The failing graft: detection and management. Semin Vasc Surg

1993; 6: 75–140.

10. Veith FV, Grapton SK, Ascer E et al. Six-year prospective multi-centre randomized trial of autogenous saphenous vein and expanded PTFE grafts in infra-inguinal arterial reconstruction. J Vasc Surg 1986; 3: 104–114.

11. Brewster DC, LaSalle AJ, Robinson JG et al. Factors affecting patency of femoro-popliteal grafts. Surg Gynecol Obstet 1983; 157: 437–442.

12. Harris PL, How TV, Jones DR. Prospective randomized clinical trial to compare in situ and reversed saphenous vein grafts for femoro-popliteal bypass. Br J Surg 1987; 74: 252–255.

13. LoGerfo FW, Quist WC, Nowak MD et al. Downstream anastomosis hyperplasia. A mechanism of failure of Dacron arterial grafts. Ann Surg 1983; 197: 479–483.

14. Sottiurai VS, Yao JST, Flinn WR et al. Intimal hyperplasia and neo-intima: an ultrastructural analysis of thrombosed grafts in humans. Surgery 1983; 93: 809–812.

15. Davies MG, Hagen PO. Pathophysiology of vein graft failures. Eur J Vasc Endovasc Surg 1995; 9: 7–18.

16. Garratt KN, Holmes DR, Bell MR et al. Restenosis after directional coronary atherectomy. J Am Coll Cardiol 1990; 16: 1165–1168.

17. Fishman DL, Leon M, Bairn DS et al. A randomized comparison of coronary stent placement and balloon angioplasty in the treatment of coronary artery disease. N Engl J Med 1994; 331: 496–501.

18. Serruys PW, de Jacques P, Kiemenyi F et al. A comparison of balloon expandable stent implantation with balloon angioplasty in patients with coronary disease. N Engl J Med 1994; 331: 489–495.

19. Schofield JP, Caskey CT. Non-viral approaches to gene therapy. Br Med Bull 1995; 51: 56–71.

20. Smith AE. Viral vectors in gene therapy. Annu Rev Microbiol 1995; 49: 807–838.

21. Vile RG, Russell SJ. Retroviruses as vectors. Br Med Bull 1995; 51: 12–30.

22. Kremer EJ, Perricaudet M. Adenovirus and adeno-associated virus mediated gene transfer. Br Med Bull 1995; 51: 31–44.

23. Yla-Herttuala S, Martin JF. Cardiovascular gene therapy. Lancet 2000; 355: 213–222.

24. Laitinen M, Pakkanen T, Donetti E et al. Gene transfer into the carotid artery using an adventitial collar: comparison of the effectiveness of the plasmid-liposome complexes, retroviruses, pseudotyped retroviruses, and adenoviruses. Hum Gene Ther 1997; 8: 1645–1650.

25. Laitinen M, Zachary I, Breier G et al. VEGF gene transfer reduces intimal thickening via increased production of nitric oxide in carotid arteries. Hum Gene Ther 1997; 8: 1737–1744.

26. Isner JM, Walsh K, Symes J et al. Arterial gene therapy for therapeutic angiogenesis in patients with peripheral artery disease. Circulation 1995; 91: 2687–2692.

27. Baumgartner I, Pieczek A, Manor O et al. Constitutive expression of phVEGF$_{165}$ after intramuscular gene transfer promotes collateral vessel development in patients with critical limb ischaemia. Circulation 1998; 97: 1114–1123.

28. Isner JM, Pieczek A, Schainfeld R et al. Clinical evidence of angiogenesis after arterial gene transfer of phVEGF$_{165}$ in patient with ischaemic limb. Lancet 1996; 348: 370–374.

29. Isner JM. Vascular Genetics Incorporated, USA. [Trial in progress]

30. RPR Gencell, USA. [Trial in progress]

31. Collateral Therapeutics Incorporation and Schering AG, Europe. [Trial in progress]

32. Isner JM, Baumgartner I, Rauh G et al. Treatment of thromboangiitis obliterans (Buerger's disease) by intramuscular gene transfer of vascular endothelial growth factor: preliminary clinical results. J Vasc Surg 1998; 28: 964–973.

33. Makinen K, Laitinen M, Manninen H, Matsi P, Alhava E, Yla-Herttuala S. Catheter-mediated VEGF gene transfer to human lower limb arteries after PTA. Circulation 1999; 100: I-1171.

34. Laitinen M, Makinen K, Manninen H et al. Adenovirus-mediated gene transfer to lower limb arteries of patients with chronic critical leg ischaemia. Hum Gene Ther 1998; 9: 1481–1486.

35. Gibbons GH, Dzau VJ. Molecular therapies for vascular diseases. Science 1996; 272: 689–693.

36. Mann MJ, Whittemore AD, Donaldson MC et al. Ex-vivo gene therapy of human vascular bypass grafts with E2F decoy: the PREVENT single-centre, randomised, controlled trial. Lancet 1999; 354: 1493–1498.

37. Grossman M, Rader DJ, Muller DMW et al. A pilot study of ex vivo gene therapy for homozygous familial hypercholesterolaemia. Nat Med 1995; 1: 1148–1154.

38. Miller N, Vile R. Targeted vectors for gene therapy. FASEB J 1995; 9: 190–199.

39. Yee J-K, Miyanohara A, LaPorte P, Bouic K, Burns JC, Friedmann T. A general method for the generation of high-titre, pantropic retroviral vectors: highly efficient infection of primary hepatocytes. Proc Natl Acad Sci USA 1994; 91: 9564–9568.

40. Burcin MM, Schiedner G, Kochanek S, Tsai SY, O'Malley BW. Adenovirus-mediated regulable target gene expression in vivo. Proc Natl Acad Sci USA 1999; 96: 355–360.

41. Stephan DJ, Yang Z-Y, San H et al. A new cationic liposome DNA complex enhances the efficiency of arterial gene transfer in vivo. Hum Gene Ther 1996; 7: 1803–1812.

42. Plank C, Mechtler K, Szoka Jr FC, Wagner E. Activation of the complement system by synthetic DNA complexes: a potential barrier for intravenous gene delivery. Hum Gene Ther 1996; 7: 1437–1446.

43. Turunen MP, Hiltunen MO, Ruponen M et al. Efficient adventitial gene delivery to rabbit carotid artery with cationic polymer-plasmid complexes. Gene Ther 1999; 6: 6–11.

Gene therapy in peripheral vascular disease

Jeff Stamatakis   James Aitken
Jenifer Smith   Michael Thompson

CHAPTER 8

What can we learn from colorectal cancer audits?

Since the UK National Health Service (NHS) reforms of 1989, there has been an insatiable appetite for measuring outcomes of treatment, the implication being that poor outcomes are due to substandard care. Audit is the only means by which clinical outcomes can be measured and it is likely to underpin the new initiative of clinical governance. If performance is to be judged on the basis of audit, it is essential that clinicians understand its nature, its pitfalls and weaknesses. It is equally important to recognise that audit has the potential to contribute far more to healthcare than just comparison of outcomes and frequently raises more questions than answers. Observed differences in survival between and within regions may be due to differing disease stage at presentation (vide infra) rather than differences between the performance of clinicians and are probably related to socio-economic status and deprivation within the patient population.[1,2]

In the early 1990s, colorectal cancer audits commenced in the English health regions of Wessex, Trent, and Wales and in the Scottish health districts of Lothian and Borders.[3–5] The authors were involved in establishing, organising and analysing these audits and there has been a substantial interchange of ideas and a joint publication.[6]

This chapter illustrates, with representative examples, some of the problems of data collection and interpretation of these large, regional audits. The principles are applicable to surgical audits in general. The chapter is in two sections, the first of which covers data collection, including the problem of imprecise definitions, and the second deals with data analysis. Difficulties produced by case-mix are referred to in each section.

Mr Jeff Stamatakis MS FRCS, Consultant Colorectal and General Surgeon, Princess of Wales Hospital, Bridgend, UK
Mr James Aitken MBBS FRCS FCS(SA) FRACS, Senior Lecturer, University of Western Australia, Australia
Dr Jenifer Smith MBBS, Director, South and West Cancer Intelligence Unit, Winchester, UK
Mr Michael Thompson MD FRCS, Department of Surgery, Queen Alexandra Hospital, Cosham, Portsmouth PO6 3LY, UK (for correspondence)

DATA COLLECTION

Accurate, reliable data, in which clinicians have confidence, are an absolute prerequisite and demand organised and disciplined methods of collection. Reported data have to be precise and detailed enough to withstand robust, and potentially hostile, scrutiny. Audit has been described as 'scientifically sloppy' with standards less stringent than those associated with research.[7] Data from audit will never be as accurate as those from research where randomisation reduces case-mix bias and precise definitions introduce a degree of control unobtainable in audit. The quality and scope of audit data will have to be greatly improved before they can be safely used to compare the performance of clinicians. In spite of this, data will be used for clinical governance and resource_allocation in the absence of other methods of achieving this and surgeons should strive to ensure data are recorded as accurately as possible.

High quality audit is resource intensive and requires extra funds. The initial costs of colorectal cancer audit were similar in each of the Regional studies, approximately £40–50 per patient. This represents less than 1% of the total treatment costs. However, successful audit also requires dedicated time from senior clinicians and resources for sophisticated statistical analysis and dissemination of the results.

DEFINITION OF POPULATION AUDITED

Comparative audit must include all patients with colorectal cancer and not omit groups such as those not having surgery or not admitted to hospital. When all cases of colorectal cancer are collected in a defined geographic population, wide variations are found in the proportion of patients submitted to surgery. For example, in the Wales and Trent audit, the non-operation rate among hospitals varied between 4% and 22% and the resection rate, for rectal cancer, varied between 58% and 95%. These variations may reflect real differences in the extent of local disease or differences in thresholds for advising against surgery on the basis of infirmity or medical co-morbidity. The surest way to reduce operative complications is to carry out a less radical resection, or even to avoid surgery altogether!

Key point 1

- Audit must include all cases presenting with the disease whether receiving surgical intervention or not.

Further difficulties with comparing outcome in different patient populations are highlighted in the Eurocare[8] and Seer[9] studies, which suggest that outcome in the US is better than continental Europe which, in turn, is better than the UK. For example, age-adjusted 5-year relative survival for colorectal cancer was reported in The Netherlands as 59%, Finland 48%, England and Scotland 41% compared with 60–64% in certain areas of the US. These studies are carried out through networks of cancer registries, which collect data on all cases within a defined geographical population. However, they include a varying sample of the respective national populations and that may not be equally representative of outcome throughout the whole country. It seems unlikely that sample bias is entirely responsible for the reported variation in survival, but even if the geographic variations are real, the lack of information on stage of disease at presentation and access to care means that it is not possible to be certain as to the cause of these differences. It is possible, even likely, that the differences are due to socio-economic factors and deprivation as well as differences in healthcare.[1,2]

Key point 2
- Precise definitions are essential to ensure conformity of data collection and permit comparisons.

CURATIVE OR PALLIATIVE SURGERY?

A colorectal cancer resection may be designated as curative or palliative on the basis of the surgeon's subjective intra-operative assessment of local or metastatic disease remaining after surgery. Ensuring conformity of assessment, particularly in relation to local disease, is difficult and there may be perverse incentives since surgeons will improve their results if difficult resections are termed 'palliative' rather than 'curative'. This may only become apparent if a surgeon's palliative resections have an unusually and consistently high survival, emphasising the importance of longitudinal data collection and analysis of a spectrum of data.

In the Wessex audit,[3] documentation of curability varied between districts from 40% to 100% of resections. The proportion of cases assessed as curative, by the surgeon, ranged from 11% to 76% between districts. Uncertainty about local curability and residual intra-abdominal disease may be genuine in up to 10% of cases, but can be further resolved by histological examination of radial margins, biopsy of suspected residual disease and postoperative liver imaging. Radial margin involvement to less than 1 mm may predict local recurrence and can be used to re-categorise the curability of a resection.[10] In the Wales and Trent audit, there was a wide variation in pathologists' documentation of lateral margin involvement of rectal specimens (8–78%, median 58%).[11]

DEFINITION OF STAGE OF DISEASE

In the UK, Dukes' classification[12] is still the most common staging for bowel cancer and there is a reluctance to change to the TNM system.[13] Precision about pathological case-mix could be improved by more accurate staging. For example, Dukes' stage C encompasses a large spectrum of disease, but attempts to make it more homogenous by division into sub-categories[14,15] have resulted in difficulties in comparing outcomes between different series. Dukes is reputed to have excluded the surgeon's operative observations in his classification as he knew how inaccurate this could be, particularly in relation to liver metastases. The original Dukes' classification was, therefore, based entirely on pathological examination of the level of invasion in a resected specimen. The importance of this is that a patient with liver metastases might have a strict pathological classification of Dukes' stage A, B or C, but a very different expected survival from the mean. In spite of Dukes' concerns about the accuracy of surgeons' observations it is now common practice to combine pathological staging with clinical assessment. Turnbull,[16] who defined Dukes' stage D as any patient with metastatic or residual local disease, first introduced this clinicopathological staging. Others have defined Dukes' stage D as any metastatic disease in the abdomen alone, as in the Wessex audit,[3] or any systemic or residual local disease, as in the Wales and Trent audit.[4] Such variation in definition makes comparison between audits difficult. The use of increasingly sophisticated pre- and intra-operative liver imaging will inevitably mean that Dukes' stage D will no longer be based on clinical assessment alone. Intensive imaging will down-stage cancers and the associated stage-migration, known as the Will Rodgers effect,[17] can make it impossible to compare outcomes between different centres.

'Stage-migration' may heavily bias outcome,[17] not least because disease-stage may have a greater impact on outcome than clinical or surgical intervention. The percentage of Dukes' A+B cancers in the Wessex audit varied between districts from 37–56% with a reciprocal gradient in the percentage of Dukes' stage D and a corresponding variation in the crude 5-year survival from 36% to 52% (Fig. 8.1). In Wales, the range of incidence in Dukes' D cancer between hospitals was 10–42%. These data suggest the extent of disease at presentation is the dominant factor in determining survival rather than differences in the access to or effectiveness of treatment.

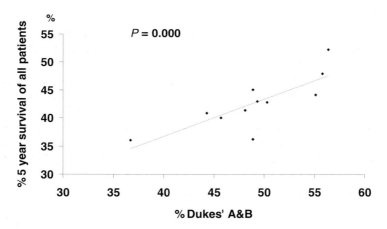

Fig. 8.1 Shows the linear correlation between case-mix as determined by the percentage of Dukes' A and B tumours in each district and the crude 5-year survival of a total population audited in each of the corresponding districts.

IMPORTANCE AND MEASUREMENT OF MEDICAL CO-MORBIDITY

The powerful effect of medical co-morbidity provides clinicians with an incentive to record all associated disease adversely affecting outcome. The

New York State Department of Health Cardiac Surgery Reporting System reported a dramatic increase in the number of recorded co-morbid risk factors following publication of the first year's report.[18] There were also anecdotal reports that high-risk patients were denied surgery. Outcome data cannot be correctly interpreted without correcting for pre-operative morbidity. All three colorectal audits[3-5] attempted to record the American Society of Anesthesiology grading (ASA), a simple but crude measure of pre-existing morbidity, but the data were very incomplete. POSSUM scores[19] can provide a more objective measure of morbidity, but require substantially more data and validation has not been uniform in the UK.[20]

EMERGENCY ADMISSION OR OPERATION?

Emergency surgery is an important factor in determining postoperative death and long-term survival in colorectal cancer. However, the precise definition of emergency surgery is critical. Many patients who have an emergency admission do not have emergency surgery and their risk of dying from surgery approximates to that of an elective case (Table 8.1). The postoperative mortality of a true emergency case is 4 times that of an elective operation[3] and it is, therefore, important that emergency should refer to surgery rather than the mode of admission. As with other case-mix factors, there was a wide variation in emergency surgery rate among hospitals. In the Wales audit this ranged between 7.5% and 32% (median 21%); this has obvious implications when comparing postoperative mortality between hospitals.

MEASUREMENT OF LOCAL RECURRENCE FOLLOWING SURGERY FOR RECTAL CANCER

The intensity of follow-up and associated investigations, which might include clinical examination only or imaging with diagnostic biopsies, will influence the detection rate of local recurrence.

Strategies for follow-up after colorectal cancer surgery vary widely and there was no consensus as to best practice among surgeons in the Wales Trent audit.[21] In these audits approximately half the patients were followed-up by their general practitioner. Few GPs have the time, confidence or expertise to accurately detect pelvic recurrence following anterior resection and it is unlikely that accurate measurement can be achieved outside a research setting.

MEASUREMENT OF DEATH FROM COLORECTAL CANCER

Imprecise recording of cause of death and recurrence of cancer leads to incomparable reporting and analysis of survival. In order to determine whether a patient died with their cancer, as a result of their cancer or with their cancer in remission requires detailed and complete individual patient data. Unfortunately, death certificates are not sufficiently accurate to determine whether cancer was the specific cause of death and analyses are normally based on the less satisfactory measure of overall survival. It is probable that data on the presence of recurrent disease and disease status at the time of death can reliably be achieved only through hospital follow-up. This is becoming

Table 8.1 The postoperative mortality by site of disease and mode of admission and operation in the Wessex colorectal audit

Site	Elective admissions and operations			Emergency admissions								
				Emergency operations			Elective operations			All operations		
	Post-operative mortality		95% CI	Post-operative mortality		95% CI	Post-operative mortality		95% CI	Post-operative mortality		95% CI
	Nos	%		Nos	%		Nos	%		Nos	%	
Rectum and sigmoid	102/2166	4.7	3.8–5.6	47/217	21.7	16.2–27.1	42/269	15.6	11.3–20.0	89/486	18.3	14.9–21.8
Proximal cancers	59/923	5.6	4.2–7.1	53/255	20.8	15.8–25.8	38/328	11.6	8.1–15.1	91/583	15.6	12.7–18.6

Table 8.2 Colostomy rates following elective surgery in patients having curative resections for rectal cancer by specialists and non-specialists in the Wessex audit

	Specialists (n = 414)		Non-specialists (n = 298)	
	%	(95% CI)	%	(95% CI)
Abdominal perineal	24	(20–28)	28	(23–33)
Anterior resection	64	(59–68)	59	(54–65)
Hartmanns	2	(1–4)	4	(2–6)
Other	10	(7–13)	9	(5–12)
Temporary stomas (anterior resection only)	57.9*	(51–64)	27.6**	(21–35)

*154 temporary colostomies out of 266 patients
**50 temporary colostomies out of 181 patients

increasingly restricted as its uncertain cost-benefit is encouraging the discharge of patients to the care of their GP. Paradoxically, some surgeons may find little incentive for pursuing follow-up, imaging or post-mortems, as these may identify unsuspected cancer recurrence. Standard follow-up protocols and methods of analysis should be agreed at the outset of any audit.

Five-year survival rates will be affected by non-cancer factors such as the age and life expectancy of the patient reflected by the background death rate within that community caused by, for example, respiratory and cardiovascular disease. For comparative purposes, 5-year survival should be standardised for age and adjusted for background mortality by calculation of the age-adjusted relative survival rates.[22]

SPECIALIST AND HIGH VOLUME SURGEONS

In both the Trent/Wales and the Wessex population audits, a small subset of patients with Dukes' C colon and rectal carcinomas, having curative, elective resections, had apparent improved overall survival rate after treatment by a specialist surgeon. However, firm conclusions cannot be drawn as there was no risk-adjusted analysis for medical co-morbidity and Dukes' C stage encompasses a wide spectrum of disease. In the Lothian and Borders audit (minimum follow-up 26 months) it has not been possible to show any inter-surgeon variation or advantage to high volume or specialist surgeons. The Wales/Trent audit also failed to show that high volume surgeons achieve a better outcome. As there are no nationally recognised definitions on what constitutes a specialist or high volume surgeon, any cut-off point is arbitrary.

Avoidance of a permanent stoma greatly affects the quality of life after rectal surgery. However, in the Wessex audit, no difference was seen between specialists and non-specialists after curative elective rectal cancer surgery. There was, however, a significantly greater use of temporary stomas after anterior resection by specialists (Table 8.2).

DATA ANALYSIS

MINIMUM AUDITABLE CASELOAD

Wide year-on-year variation of outcome is a well-documented phenomenon[23–25] within comparatively small datasets. This can result in considerable differences in outcomes achieved by different surgeons within a single year, which disappear with time as increasing numbers of patients are audited as shown in the Lothian audit in Figure 8.2. The total number of patients studied must be large enough to even out short-term fluctuations of less common adverse events. The Cardiac Surgery Reporting System only included surgeons who recruited 200 relevant cases. The minimum number of colorectal cancer patients required for reliable individual comparisons is dependent on the frequency of the adverse event studied. For many purposes 150 cases is probably sufficient, but even on this basis a surgeon resecting 20 colorectal cancers per year could only have his or her postoperative mortality assessed after 8–10 years. If a third of these cases were rectal cancers, it would take over 30 years to recruit sufficient cases for reliable surgeon specific

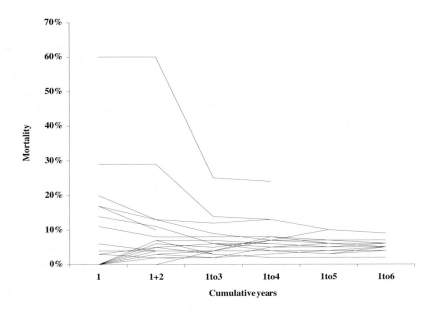

Fig. 8.2 The Lothian audit for colorectal cancer. The cumulative associated mortality for individual surgeons over a 6-year period. Large initial differences between surgeons disappear over the 6-year period.

survival analysis. There is a lack of consensus as to what constitutes a high volume surgeon. For example, a recent study of curative rectal cancer surgery[26] showed that surgeons carrying out more than 21 resections in the 8-year study had better outcomes. This caseload scarcely reflects high volume. With increasing numbers of colorectal surgeons, individuals will recruit a smaller number of cases and this is one reason for analysis to be unit rather than surgeon-based.

Key point 3 & 4

- Raw audit data, not corrected for risk factors, is of little value in comparative audit.

- Social and economic deprivation may have a significant effect on outcome yet is not routinely recorded at patient level.

COMPARING OUTCOMES AND RISK STRATIFICATION

All audit is comparative, whether amongst contributing colleagues, other institutions, or external guidelines. However, the ranking of performance in league tables using raw audit data, can be misleading. These colorectal cancer audits have demonstrated wide regional variations in many risk factors that influence outcome after colorectal cancer surgery. Several studies have demonstrated the difference between observed and expected outcome when adjustment is made for case-mix.[27] Case-mix adjustment is an inexact science that may not be reproducible. The Cardiac Surgery Reporting System only included uncomplicated coronary artery bypass surgery and used 40 well-established cardiac risk factors to adjust for the single outcome measure of mortality. Despite this extensive standardisation, some surgeons operating in different hospitals had substantially different risk-adjusted mortality rates. This suggests that other variable(s) were influencing outcome. Regional variations in deprivation scores appear to be a very important independent, significant, factor in cancer outcomes.[2]

INTERPRETATION OF RESULTS TO DATE

These regional colorectal audits[3–5] have been able to determine average values and ranges for a number of processes, procedures and outcomes amongst practising surgeons. These may be used as very crude benchmarks for the main clinical outcomes such as postoperative mortality, anastomotic leak rates, stoma rates, local recurrence and 5-year survival after colorectal cancer surgery. They have also determined the average time lag to diagnosis and treatment achieved with existing resources. These results have been used to set standards against which surgeons can compare their own results.[28] However, it is important to consider the confidence intervals, both for the standards against which comparisons are to be made and for the results of local audits, before determining whether differences in outcome are statistically significant. The confidence intervals will be wide if the numbers are small and it may not be possible to conclude, even with large differences in outcomes, that these are statistically significant. In order to draw conclusions about the performance of an individual surgeon, it is essential to ensure that like is being compared to like and to use risk-adjustment to evaluate differences between observed and expected outcomes.

Key point 5

- The use of a national database, such as that devised by the Association of Coloproctology of Great Britain and Ireland for colorectal cancer which includes information appropriate for risk modelling, will be of value in comparative audit and clinical governance.

THE ASSOCIATION OF COLOPROCTOLOGY OF GREAT BRITAIN AND IRELAND DATASET AND DATABASE

Lessons learnt from these colorectal cancer audits, some of which are set out above, acted as the stimulus to produce a minimum data set[29] which may help to overcome some, but not all, of the pitfalls in data collection for colorectal cancer audit. Fundamental to the data set is a data dictionary, which precisely defines each field to ensure conformity of interpretation. The Society of Cardiothoracic Surgeons of Great Britain and Ireland has used an agreed data set for some years and publishes an annual report, including risk stratification analysis, which permits comparative audit of outcomes.[30]

Patients have a right to know that clinicians' performance is under scrutiny and that they are receiving a professionally agreed standard of care. Doctors do not expect airline safety announcements to include their pilot's last score in the flight simulator, but they do expect pilots to remain under regular review and to be retrained if they do not meet an agreed standard. Increasingly, surgeons will find their individual performance under close scrutiny and it is in their own interest to demonstrate that they take a lead role in the recording and analysis of data that may determine their professional future.

Key points for clinical practice

- Audit must include all cases presenting with the disease whether receiving surgical intervention or not.

- Precise definitions are essential to ensure conformity of data collection and permit comparisons.

- Raw audit data, not corrected for risk factors, is of little value in comparative audit.

- Social and economic deprivation may have a significant effect on outcome yet is not routinely recorded at patient level.

- The use of a national database, such as that devised by the Association of Coloproctology of Great Britain and Ireland for colorectal cancer which includes information appropriate for risk modelling, will be of value in comparative audit and clinical governance.

References

1. Coleman MP, Babb P, Damiecki P et al. Cancer survival trends in England and Wales. 1971–1995; Deprivation and NHS region. Series Studies on medical and population subjects. Office for National Statistics No.61. London: The Stationery Office, 1999.
2. Monnet E, Boutron MC, Faivre J, Milan C. Influence of socioeconomic status on prognosis of colorectal cancer. Cancer 1993; 72: 1165–1170.
3. Wessex Colorectal Cancer Audit. First Report May 1993. Wessex Cancer Intelligence Unit, Highcroft, Romsey Road, Winchester SO2 5DH, UK.
4. Mella J, Biffin A, Radcliffe AG, Stamatakis JD, Steele RJC. Population-based audit of colorectal cancer management in two health regions. Br J Surg 1997; 84: 1731–1736.
5. The Lothian and Borders Large Bowel Cancer Project. The immediate outcome of surgery. Br J Surg 1995; 82: 888–890.
6. Aitken RJ, Thompson MR, Radcliffe AG, Stamatakis J, Steele RJC. Training in colorectal cancer surgery. Observations from three UK prospective regional audits. BMJ 1999; 318: 702–703.
7. Smith R. Audit and research. BMJ 1992: 305: 905–906.
8. Gatta G, Faivre J, Capocaccia R, Ponz de Leon M, and EUROCARE Working Group. Survival of colorectal cancer patients in Europe during the period 1978–1989. Eur J Cancer 1998; 34: 2176–2183.
9. National Cancer Institute SEER Stat – cancer incidence public use database. 1973–95. Release 1.1 Bethesda, MD: National Cancer Institute, 1998.
10. Adam IJ, Mohamdee MO, Martin IG et al. Role of circumferential margin involvement in the local recurrence of rectal cancer. Lancet 1994; 344: 707–711.
11. Bull AD, Biffin AHB, Mella J et al. Colorectal cancer pathology reporting: a regional audit. J Clin Pathol 1997; 50: 138–142.

12. Dukes CE. The classification of cancer of the rectum. J Pathol Bacteriol 1932; 35: 323–332.
13. UICC Committee on TNM Classification. Malignant tumours of the Oesophagus, Stomach, Colon and Rectum. Geneva: International Union Against Cancer, 1966.
14. Gabriel WB, Dukes CE, Bussey HJR. Lymphatic spread in cancer of the rectum. Br J Surg 1935; 23: 309–320.
15. Astler VB, Coller FA. The prognostic significance of direct extension of carcinoma of the colon and rectum. Ann Surg 1954; 139: 846–852.
16. Turnbull Jr RB, Kyle K, Watson FR, Spratt J. Cancer of the colon: the influence of the no-touch isolation technique on survival rates. Ann Surg 1967; 166: 420–427.
17 Feinstein AR, Sosin DM, Wells CK. The Will Rodgers phenomenon: stage migration and new diagnostic techniques as a source of misleading statistics for survival in cancer. N Engl J Med 1985; 312: 1604–1608.
18. Schneider EC, Epstein AM. Influence of cardiac surgery performance reports on referral practice and access to care. A survey of cardiovascular specialists. N Engl J Med 1996; 335: 251–256.
19. Copeland GP, Sagar P, Brennan M et al. Risk-adjusted analysis of surgeon performance: a 1 year study. Br J Surg 1995; 82 :408–411.
20. Prytherch DR, Whiteley MS, Higgins B, Weaver PC Prout WG, Powell SJ. Possum and Portsmouth Possum for predicting mortality. Physiological and Operative Severity Score for the enumeration of mortality and morbidity. Br J Surg 1998; 85: 1217–1220.
21. Mella J, Datta SN, Biffin A, Radcliffe AG, Steele RJ, Stamatakis JD. Surgeon's follow-up practice after resection of colorectal cancer. Ann R Coll Surg Engl 1997; 79: 206–209.
22. Hakulinen T, Abeywikrama K. A computer program package for relative survival analysis. Comp Prog Biomed 1987; 19: 197–207.
23. Poloniecki J, Valencia O, Littlejohns P. Cumulative risk adjusted mortality chart for detecting changes in death rate; observational study of heart surgery. BMJ 1998; 316: 1697–1700.
24. Marson LP, Stevenson J, Gould A, Aitken RJ. Intersurgeon variation following colorectal cancer surgery appears to decrease with progressive audit. Br J Surg 1997: 84 (Suppl): 24.
25. Parry GJ, Gould CR, McCabe CJ, Tarnow-Mordi WO. Annual league tables of mortality in neonatal intensive care units; longitudinal study. BMJ 1998; 316: 1931–1935.
26. Porter GA, Soskolne CL, Yakimets WW, Newman SC. Surgeon related factors and outcome in rectal cancer. Ann Surg 1998; 227: 157–167.
27. Sagar PM, Hartley MN, Mancey-Jones B, Sedman PC, May J, MacFie J. Comparative audit of colorectal resection with the POSSUM scoring system. Br J Surg. 1994; 81: 1492–1494.
28. The Royal College of Surgeons of England and Association of Coloproctology of Great Britain and Ireland. Guidelines for the management of Colorectal Cancer. London: The Royal College of Surgeons of England, 1996.
29. www.cancernw.org/clinit/products_acp.htm
30. The Society of Cardiothoracic Surgeons of Great Britain and Ireland National Cardiac Surgical Database Report 1998. May 1999.

Marion Jonas   John H. Scholefield

Anal fissure and chemical sphincterotomy

Anal fissure is a linear tear in the lining of the distal anal canal below the dentate line. It is a common condition affecting all age groups, but is seen particularly in young and otherwise healthy adults, with equal incidence across the sexes. The classical symptoms are of anal pain during or after defaecation accompanied by the passage of bright red blood per anus. The pain is often severe and may last for a few minutes during, or persist for several hours after, defaecation; bleeding is separate from the stool and usually modest. In addition, pruritus ani may accompany up to 50% of anal fissures. Symptoms from fissures cause considerable morbidity and reduction in quality of life.[1]

On examination the fissure may be apparent as the buttocks are parted, but marked spasm of the anal sphincter often obscures the view. An early fissure, if seen, has sharply demarcated, fresh mucosal edges and there may be granulation tissue in its base. With increasing chronicity the margins of the fissure become indurated and there is a distinct lack of granulation tissue. Horizontal fibres of the internal sphincter muscle may be evident in the base of a chronic fissure and secondary changes such as a sentinel skin tag, hypertrophied anal papilla or a degree of anal stenosis are often present.

The majority of anal fissures are probably acute and relatively short-lived, resolving either spontaneously or with simple dietary modification to increase fibre, and stool-softening laxatives where appropriate. The distinction between acute and chronic fissures is somewhat arbitrary and cannot be made reliably solely on appearance. However, the accepted definition is that fissures failing to heal within 6 weeks despite straightforward dietary measures are designated as 'chronic'.

Ms Marion Jonas FRCS, Research Fellow, Section of Surgery, University Hospital, Queen's Medical Centre, E Floor, West Block, Nottingham NG7 2UH, UK (for correspondence)
Prof. John H. Scholefield FRCS ChM, Professor of Surgery, Section of Surgery, University Hospital, Queen's Medical Centre, E Floor, West Block, Nottingham NG7 2UH, UK

Although a proportion (10–30%) of chronic fissures will eventually resolve with conservative measures, most require further intervention in order to heal. Fissures are usually single and in the posterior midline, but 10% of women and 1% of men have anterior fissures. Women with symptoms following childbirth account for 3–11% of all chronic fissures and tend to have anterior fissures.[2] Multiple fissures or those in a lateral position on the anal margin may indicate underlying inflammatory bowel disease, syphilis, or immunosuppression. However, it should be recognised that most fissures occurring in the presence of inflammatory bowel disease are in the posterior midline and at least one-half are also painful. Fissures that are resistant to treatment should prompt further investigation including examination under anaesthesia and appropriate biopsy.

Chronic anal fissures are generally associated with raised resting anal canal pressure, secondary to hypertonicity of the internal anal sphincter, and treatment is directed at reducing this. Traditional surgical treatments, namely manual anal dilatation or sphincterotomy, effectively heal most fissures within a few weeks, but may result in permanently impaired anal continence. This has led to the search for alternative non-surgical treatment, and various pharmacological agents have been shown to lower resting anal pressure and heal fissures without threatening anal continence.

PATHOGENESIS OF ANAL FISSURE

The pathogenesis of chronic anal fissure is ill understood. The surgical dogma is that the passage of a hard stool bolus traumatises the anal mucosa. This is a plausible initiating factor, but does not explain why only one in four patients report constipation, while symptoms may follow a bout of diarrhoea. There may be a dietary association as people taking a diet low in fibre appear to be at increased risk of developing anal fissures.[3]

Alternative theories as to the pathogenic process leading to the development of chronic fissures have been postulated.

CHILDBIRTH

Up to 11% of patients with chronic anal fissures develop symptoms following childbirth.[2] The risk increases with traumatic deliveries and the fissures are commonly in the anterior midline. Shearing forces from the fetal head on the anal mucosa, and tethering of the anal mucosa to underlying muscle postpartum thereby rendering it more susceptible to trauma, have been suggested as possible precipitating factors. However, both are speculative theories of the aetiology of anal fissure and difficult to substantiate. Interestingly, women with postpartum fissures tend not to display raised resting anal canal pressures, and endoanal ultrasonography may demonstrate thinning or disruption of the internal anal sphincter.

INTERNAL ANAL SPHINCTER HYPERTONIA

The resting pressure in the anal canal is largely a function of the internal sphincter which has intrinsic tone that is both nerve-mediated via α-adrenergic pathways and inherently myogenic. Relaxation of this smooth muscle occurs automatically in response to rectal distension, the so-called rectoanal inhibitory reflex. Acetylcholine via muscarinic receptors and β-adrenergic stimulation both mediate relaxation in vitro;[4] electrical field stimulation also causes relaxation and nitric oxide (NO) has been identified as the neurotransmitter responsible.[5]

Patients with chronic anal fissures generally have raised resting anal pressures due to hypertonicity of the internal anal sphincter, but the causative mechanisms are unclear.[6] A long high pressure zone in the anal canal and ultra-slow waves are seen more frequently in fissure patients than in healthy controls and there may be an abnormal rectoanal inhibitory reflex.[6] Pharmacological agents that relax the internal anal sphincter, and surgical procedures which stretch (manual anal dilatation) or incise it (sphincterotomy), reduce anal canal pressure and lead to healing in the majority of chronic fissures. Drugs appear to have a reversible effect on the internal anal sphincter muscle: resting anal pressures return to pre-treatment values even after a fissure has healed, suggesting that internal sphincter hypertonia may predate the onset of a fissure.[7] Furthermore, the anal spasm is probably not a response to pain as topical local anaesthetic alleviates the discomfort but does not reduce the spasm.[8]

LOCAL ISCHAEMIA

Chronic anal fissure has been described as an ischaemic ulcer. The distal anal canal receives its blood supply from the inferior rectal arteries, branches of the internal pudendal arteries. Angiography of the inferior rectal vessels in cadavers has demonstrated a paucity of arterioles at the posterior commissure of the anal canal, the site for which fissures have a predilection, in 85% of cases.[9,10] Blood flow to the distal anal canal, measured by laser Doppler flowmetry, is inversely correlated with anal pressure, increasing as pressures fall. General anaesthesia, sphincterotomy, and the application of topical glyceryl trinitrate (GTN) ointment all lower resting anal pressure and simultaneously increase the local blood flow in the distal anal canal of patients with anal fissure.[11,12] As lateral internal sphincterotomy and topical GTN successfully heal approximately 95% and 65% of fissures, respectively, the local blood supply prior to treatment may have been inadequate for healing to occur.[13–15] Blood vessels traversing the hypertonic internal sphincter en route to the anal mucosa may be compressed, compromising perfusion locally. Anal spasm in patients with chronic anal fissures appears to predate the fissure; this supports an ischaemic basis for chronic fissure, and implies that some people may be predisposed towards developing an anal fissure, or at risk of delayed healing once a fissure has occurred.[12]

Histological examination of biopsies of internal anal sphincter taken both from the base of chronic fissures and at sites remote from it demonstrated fibrosis in all regions,[16] leading to the hypothesis that an underlying inflammatory process is present, myositis being followed by fibrosis. However, the fibrosis itself may be secondary to ischaemia.

Anti-endothelial cell antibodies (AECAs) identified in the sera of patients with chronic anal fissure may indicate an autoimmune process.[17] Circulating autoantibodies may activate endothelium, while activated endothelial cells may express antigens and induce the formation of autoantibodies. The aetiology of a primary insult to the endothelium is not known, but it is conceivable that AECAs may be responsible for amplifying pre-existing vascular damage. Vasoactive autacoids produced by activated endothelium can cause vasoconstriction which may precipitate or exacerbate local ischaemia. Furthermore, endothelial dysfunction is characterized by reduced NO synthesis, and so the success of NO donors as treatment for chronic fissures may support the suggestion of an autoimmune pathogenesis.

Despite various theories, however, the pathogenesis of chronic anal fissure remains uncertain.

TREATMENT

ACUTE FISSURE

Over 90% of acute anal fissures are short-lived, healing spontaneously or with simple measures. A high fibre diet with increased intake of water is recommended, stool softening laxatives where required, and warm sitz baths for symptomatic relief. Topical hydrocortisone and local anaesthetics probably confer no added benefit over dietary bran, and may even be detrimental.[18] In one study, topical steroids precipitated extensive anal herpes, previously occult, in a patient with anal fissure.[18] Topical local anaesthetic appears to delay healing when compared with bran supplements or topical hydrocortisone, and skin sensitisation may develop.[18] Lubricated anal dilators, popular for a while, fell out of favour as studies reported a high relapse rate.

CHRONIC FISSURE

The majority of long-standing, chronic fissures require additional intervention in order to heal. These patients generally have raised resting anal pressures, and treatment is directed at reducing the spasm of the internal anal sphincter.

Traditional surgical procedures, manual anal dilatation or internal sphincterotomy, carry the risk of irreversible impairment of anal continence. Various pharmacological agents have been shown to lower resting anal pressure and promote fissure healing, and 'chemical sphincterotomy' is now the accepted first line treatment in many centres.

Organic nitrates
Recognition of NO as the non-adrenergic, non-cholinergic neurotransmitter mediating relaxation of the internal anal sphincter has initiated the widespread use of organic nitrates in the treatment of chronic anal fissure. These agents are metabolised at a cellular level to release NO which, in turn, mediates relaxation of the internal sphincter via the guanylyl cyclase pathway by increasing cGMP levels within the smooth muscle cells.

Preparations of isosorbide dinitrate and GTN have been used with success, most studies reporting healing in the majority of cases.[13,14,19,20] Topical GTN ointment applied to the anal verge is generally accepted as an effective treatment for chronic fissures. However, there is confusion over the optimal dose required: the dose of GTN administered depends upon both the concentration and volume of ointment applied. Other factors affecting absorption such as the precise site of application (perianal skin or anal canal), and the vehicle used to deliver GTN to the area are also likely to be important. A regimen using a 'pea-sized amount', (approximately 0.5 g), of 0.2% GTN ointment applied 2–3 times daily to the distal anal canal for up to 8 weeks, has been shown to heal two-thirds of chronic fissures, but over one-half of these patients develop headaches as a side effect of the treatment.[13,14,21,22] Although usually mild, transient and tolerable, often diminishing in intensity and duration with continued application, the headaches may be sufficiently severe to reduce compliance or lead to cessation of treatment in some cases. Preparations containing higher concentrations of GTN usually result in an increase in the incidence and severity of headaches.[23,24] For maximal benefit in the clinical setting, topical 0.2% GTN should probably be prescribed for longer than 6 weeks and some fissures may take up to 12 weeks to heal.[22,25,26]

The long-term follow-up by questionnaire of patients participating in a randomised controlled trial where twice daily 0.2% GTN healed their chronic fissures, reported a recurrence of symptoms in 27% patients within a median of 2 years: over two-thirds of these resolved with further GTN.[27] Treatment with GTN seems to be as effective for recurrent as for primary fissures.

Key point 3
- Pharmacological agents which effectively cause a 'chemical sphincterotomy' heal the majority of fissures. Topical 0.2% glyceryl trinitrate ointment is probably the most widely used first line treatment in the UK, but many patients experience troublesome headaches on this therapy and alternative treatments are currently under investigation.

Calcium channel blockers

Nifedipine and diltiazem are widely prescribed in clinical practice as anti-anginal and antihypertensive agents, blocking slow L-type calcium channels in vascular smooth muscle to cause relaxation and vasodilatation. Both drugs also cause relaxation of smooth muscle cells in other tissues: nifedipine reduces lower oesophageal sphincter pressure, and recent studies have demonstrated that both nifedipine and diltiazem decrease resting anal pressure in patients with chronic anal fissure.[28,29] A prospective cohort study reported healing in 9 of 15 patients with chronic fissures treated with oral nifedipine (20 mg twice daily),[28] and a randomised multi-centre study showed benefit with topical nifedipine (0.2% twice daily) but included both acute and chronic fissures making comparative interpretation of the results difficult.

A randomised study of 40 patients has shown that oral and topical diltiazem heal chronic anal fissures. Oral diltiazem was less effective (47% healed) and caused side effects (nausea, vomiting, headache or rash) in one-third of the patients. Topical diltiazem, however, was comparable to GTN in terms of healing (71% healed) without side effects.[30] In vitro experiments on isolated sheep internal anal sphincter have shown that diltiazem has a slower onset of action than GTN but more sustained effect,[31] and in healthy volunteers, topical 2% diltiazem was reported to significantly reduce resting anal pressure for up to 5 h.[32]

Botulinum A toxin

Botulinum toxin A, produced by *Clostridium botulinum*, is a lethal biological toxin but has, nonetheless, been of enormous therapeutic value in the treatment of various ophthalmological and neurological disorders. The potent neurotoxin binds to presynaptic cholinergic nerve terminals, inhibiting the release of acetylcholine at the neuromuscular junction. When injected into the endplate zone of the muscle, paralysis occurs within hours and persists for 3–4 months, until there has been axonal regeneration.

Uncontrolled studies have reported that botulinum toxin A injection into the anal sphincter lowered resting anal pressure and healed up to 82% of chronic anal fissures, although 6% recurred within 6 months; post-injection perianal thrombosis occurred in 10% of patients, and transient faecal incontinence in 7%.[33] A randomised trial comparing botulinum toxin injection with 6 weeks of 0.2% GTN in 50 patients reported healing rates of 96% and 60%, respectively, with no adverse effects in those patients receiving botulinum toxin.[34]

There is confusion in the literature concerning the optimal site of injection of the toxin, whether external or internal anal sphincter, and the mode of action of botulinum toxin is unclear. The toxin would be expected to cause relaxation in the striated external sphincter muscle, but there are no corresponding acetylcholine receptors in the smooth muscle of the internal sphincter. In fact, acetylcholine in vitro mediates relaxation in the smooth muscle of the internal sphincter and so blockade of its release ought to increase anal tone.[4] Precise localisation of the injection site is probably difficult and it is likely that the toxin diffuses into adjacent tissue planes. It is conceivable, therefore, that the action is entirely on the striated external sphincter, thought to contribute up to 30% of resting anal pressure.[35] However, it has been reported that maximal voluntary squeeze pressures at 1 and 2 months following injection of botulinum toxin into the internal sphincter were not significantly different to pretreatment values.[34]

The treatment is advantageous in that a single injection produces a prolonged effect that is ultimately reversible, avoiding permanent injury to the anal sphincter mechanism. Unfortunately, it is invasive and complications such as perianal haematoma, sepsis, and pain during injection of the toxin may occur. On balance it is difficult to be certain about the exact injection site, and patients may find the procedure uncomfortable. Despite evidence to support its efficacy, the role of botulinum toxin in the management of chronic fissures remains unclear.

Surgery

Pharmacological agents offer useful first line treatment for chronic fissures, but failure of medical therapy and persistent symptoms warrant surgical intervention. The surgical approaches to chronic fissures have included manual anal dilation or sphincterotomy, and most recently advancement flaps to cover the mucosal defect.[36,37]

Key point 4

- Where pharmacological therapy fails or fissures recur frequently and patients have raised resting anal pressure, lateral internal sphincterotomy is the surgical treatment of choice. Complications may be avoided through careful patient selection and once the incision is limited to the length of the fissure.

Manual anal dilatation should be abandoned: it is uncontrolled and the resultant disruption to the sphincter mechanism, demonstrated by endoanal ultrasonography, may be significant. A meta-analysis of trials comparing anal dilatation and internal sphincterotomy reported sphincterotomy to be superior: healing rates are higher and impairment of continence less likely.[15] Lateral sphincterotomy is preferable to a posterior incision which takes longer to heal, is more likely to become infected, and may form a keyhole deformity in up to 28% of cases, possibly leading to imperfect closure of the anal canal or trapping of faeces and soiling.[38] There is little difference in terms of healing and complications between open and closed techniques for sphincterotomy, and the choice of anaesthesia is probably irrelevant.[15] Sphincterotomy should be limited to the length of the fissure;[39] high complication rates reported in early studies may result from extended sphincterotomy incisions. Postoperative endosonographic assessment revealed that sphincterotomy was often more extensive than appreciated at the time of operation, particularly in female patients.[40] In order to avoid complications in women, especially those with post partum fissures who may already have sustained significant damage to the anal sphincter, it is prudent to assess the integrity of the anal sphincter using anal manometry and anorectal ultrasound prior to surgical intervention. Where the internal sphincter is already compromised and resting anal pressure

---

Key point 5

- Where 'chemical sphincterotomy' fails and resting anal pressures are not raised, in women with postpartum fissures for example, an island advancement flap should be considered.

---

is not raised, it is probably better to perform an anal advancement flap to repair the mucosal defect rather than jeopardize anal continence through iatrogenic injury to the sphincter. Patients with on-going symptoms after sphincterotomy should also have anal manometry and endoanal ultrasonography to determine anal pressure and the adequacy of the previous sphincterotomy.

Key points for clinical practice

- .Anal fissures are common but most are short-lived and heal spontaneously. Those which persist and require intervention cause considerable morbidity in an otherwise healthy young population.

- Lateral internal sphincterotomy, traditionally the 'gold standard' treatment for chronic fissures, may cause a degree of anal incontinence in up to 45% of patients.

- Pharmacological agents which effectively cause a 'chemical sphincterotomy' heal the majority of fissures. Topical 0.2% glyceryl trinitrate ointment is probably the most widely used first line treatment in the UK, but many patients experience troublesome headaches on this therapy and alternative treatments are currently under investigation.

- Where pharmacological therapy fails or fissures recur frequently and patients have raised resting anal pressure, lateral internal sphincterotomy is the surgical treatment of choice. Complications may be avoided through careful patient selection and once the incision is limited to the length of the fissure.

- Where 'chemical sphincterotomy' fails and resting anal pressures are not raised, in women with postpartum fissures for example, an island advancement flap should be considered.

References

1. Sailer M, Bussen D, Debus ES, Fuchs KH, Thiede A. Quality of life in patients with benign anorectal disorders. Br J Surg 1998; 85: 1716–1719.
2. Martin JD. Postpartum anal fissure. Lancet 1953; i: 271–273.
3. Jensen SL. Diet and other risk factors for fissure-in-ano. Prospective case control study. Dis Colon Rectum 1988; 31: 770–773.

4. Burleigh DE, A DM, Parks AG. Responses of isolated human internal anal sphincter to drugs and electrical field stimulation. Gastroenterology 1979; 77: 484–490.
5. O'Kelly T, Brading A, Mortensen N. Nerve mediated relaxation of the human internal anal sphincter: the role of nitric oxide. Gut 1993; 34: 689–693.
6. Keck JO, Staniunas RJ, Coller JA, Barrett RC, Oster ME. Computer-generated profiles of the anal canal in patients with anal fissure. Dis Colon Rectum 1995; 38: 72–79.
7. Lund JN, Parsons SL, Scholefield JH. Spasm of the internal anal sphincter in anal fissure – cause or effect? Gastroenterology 1996; 110: A711.
8. Minguez M, Tomas-Ridocci M, Garcia A, Benages A. Pressure of the anal canal in patients with hemorrhoids or with anal fissure. Effect of the topical application of an anesthetic gel [in Spanish]. Rev Esp Enferm Dig 1992; 81: 103–107.
9. Lund JN, Binch C, McGrath J, Sparrow RA, Scholefield JH. Topographical distribution of blood supply to the anal canal. Br J Surg 1999; 86: 496–498.
10. Klosterhalfen B, Vogel P, Rixen H, Mittermayer C. Topography of the inferior rectal artery: a possible cause of chronic, primary anal fissure. Dis Colon Rectum 1989; 32: 43–52.
11. Schouten WR, Briel JW, Auwerda JJ. Relationship between anal pressure and anodermal blood flow. The vascular pathogenesis of anal fissures. Dis Colon Rectum 1994; 37: 664–669.
12. Lund JN, Scholefield JH. Internal sphincter spasm in anal fissure. Br J Surg 1997; 84: 1723-1724.
13. Lund JN, Scholefield JH. A randomised, prospective, double-blind, placebo-controlled trial of glyceryl trinitrate ointment in the treatment of anal fissure. Lancet 1997; 349: 11–14.
14. Carapeti EA, Kamm MA, McDonald PJ, Chadwick SJ, Melville D, Phillips RK. Randomised controlled trial shows that glyceryl trinitrate heals anal fissures, higher doses are not more effective, and there is a high recurrence rate. Gut 1999; 44: 727–730.
15. Nelson RL. Meta-analysis of operative techniques for fissure-in-ano. Dis Colon Rectum 1999; 42: 1424–1428; discussion 1428-1431.
16. Brown AC, Sumfest JM, Rozwadowski JV. Histopathology of the internal anal sphincter in chronic anal fissure. Dis Colon Rectum 1989; 32: 680–683.
17. Maria G, Brisinda D, Ruggieri MP, Civello IM, Brisinda G. Identification of anti-endothelial cell antibodies in patients with chronic anal fissure. Surgery 1999; 126: 535–540.
18. Jensen SL. Treatment of first episodes of acute anal fissure: prospective randomised study of lignocaine ointment versus hydrocortisone ointment or warm sitz baths plus bran. BMJ 1986; 292: 1167–1169.
19. Schouten WR, Briel JW, Boerma MO, Auwerda JJA. Pathophysiological aspects and clinical outcome of intra-anal application of isosorbide-dinitrate in patients with chronic anal fissure. Gut 1995; 36 (Suppl. 1): A16.
20. Lysy J, Israelit-Yatzkan Y, Sestiere-Ittah M, Keret D, Goldin E. Treatment of chronic anal fissure with isosorbide dinitrate: long-term results and dose determination. Dis Colon Rectum 1998; 41: 1406–1410.
21. Kennedy ML, Sowter S, Nguyen H, Lubowski DZ. Glyceryl trinitrate ointment for the treatment of chronic anal fissure: results of a placebo-controlled trial and long-term follow-up. Dis Colon Rectum 1999; 42: 1000-1006.
22. Dorfman G, Levitt M, Platell C. Treatment of chronic anal fissure with topical glyceryl trinitrate. Dis Colon Rectum 1999; 42: 1007-1010.
23. Lund JN, Armitage NC, Scholefield JH. The use of glyceryl trinitrate in the treatment of anal fissure: results of a pilot study. Gut 1995; 37 (Suppl. 2): A5.
24. Watson SJ, Kamm MA, Nicholls RJ, Phillips RKS. Topical glyceryl trinitrate in treatment of chronic anal fissure. Br J Surg 1996; 83: 771–775.
25. Jonas M, Lobo DN, Gudgeon AM. Lateral internal sphincterotomy is not redundant in the era of glyceryl trinitrate therapy for chronic anal fissure. J R Soc Med 1999; 92: 186–188.
26. Hasegawa H, Radley S, Morton DG, Dorricott NJ, Campbell DJ, Keighley MR. Audit of topical glyceryl trinitrate for treatment of fissure-in-ano. Ann R Coll Surg Engl 2000; 82: 27–30.
27. Lund JN, Scholefield JH. Follow-up of patients with chronic anal fissure treated with topical glyceryl trinitrate [letter]. Lancet 1998; 352: 1681.

28. Cook T, Smilgin Humphreys MM, McMortensen NJ. Oral nifedipine is an effective treatment for chronic anal fissures. Colorectal Dis 1999; 1 (Suppl. 1): 55.

29. Jonas M, Scholefield JH. Oral and topical diltiazem lower resting anal pressure in patients with chronic anal fissure. Colorectal Dis 1999; 1 (Suppl. 1): 55.

30. Jonas M, Scholefield JH. Oral and topical diltiazem are effective treatment for chronic anal fissures. Gut 2000; 46 (Suppl. 11): A83.

31. Jonas M, Wilson VG, Scholefield JH. Comparison of the effects of glyceryl trinitrate (GTN) and diltiazem on isolated sheep internal anal sphincter. Gut 2000; 46 (Suppl 11): A83.

32. Carapeti EKM, Evans BK, Phillips RKS. Topical diltiazem and bethanecol decrease anal sphincter pressure without side effects. Gut 1999; 45: 719–722.

33. Jost WH. One hundred cases of anal fissure treated with botulin toxin: early and long-term results. Dis Colon Rectum 1997; 40: 1029–1032.

34. Brisinda G, Maria G, Bentivoglio AR, Cassetta E, Gui D, Albanese A. A comparison of injections of botulinum toxin and topical nitroglycerin ointment for the treatment of chronic anal fissure [see comments]. N Engl J Med 1999; 341: 65–69.

35. Lestar B, Penninckx F, Kerremans R. The composition of anal basal pressure. An in vivo and in vitro study in man. Int J Colorectal Dis 1989; 4: 118–122.

36. Leong AF, Seow-Choen F. Lateral sphincterotomy compared with anal advancement flap for chronic anal fissure. Dis Colon Rectum 1995; 38: 69–71.

37. Nyam DCNK, Wilson RG, Stewart KJ, Farouk R, Bartolo DC. Island advancement flaps in the management of anal fissures. Br J Surg 1995; 82: 326–328.

38. Abcarian H. Surgical correction of chronic anal fissure: results of lateral internal sphincterotomy vs. fissurectomy – midline sphincterotomy. Dis Colon Rectum 1980; 23: 31–36.

39. Littlejohn DR, Newstead GL. Tailored lateral sphincterotomy for anal fissure [see comments]. Dis Colon Rectum 1997; 40: 1439–1442.

40. Sultan AH, Kamm MA, Nicholls RJ, Bartram CI. Prospective study of the extent of internal anal sphincter division during lateral sphincterotomy. Dis Colon Rectum 1994; 37: 1031–1033.

Russell W. Strong

The management of blunt liver injuries

The liver is the largest solid abdominal organ. Despite the relative protection of the overlying ribs, it is susceptible to compressive forces that can fracture the soft parenchyma. Motor vehicle accidents are the most frequent cause. There could be a greater propensity for blunt liver injuries to occur in countries where the driver occupies the right side of the vehicle than those where the driver sits on the left side. Less frequent causes of compressive injury include crushing in an industrial accident; when run over by a vehicle; trodden on by a horse; a direct blow from a blunt object and a fall from a height.

The liver may fracture in several ways. There may be multiple lacerations of varying extent and depth. With a severe injury, there may be radiating fractures from a central area of pulverised parenchyma. Central disruption of hepatic parenchyma from a compression injury may occur with or without rupture of the capsule. When the capsule remains intact, blood may be extravasated into the liver substance with the development of an intrahepatic haematoma of varying size or bleeding beneath the capsule which results in a subcapsular haematoma. Shear forces generated by rapid deceleration may cause the liver to be torn from its attachments and the hepatic veins to be avulsed from the inferior vena cava. This can occur with or without major parenchymal disruption.

Although an isolated liver injury can occur, the mechanism of blunt trauma means that it is frequently associated with other significant injuries: head, chest, orthopaedic and other intra-abdominal organs. These may mask the liver injury which can be difficult to diagnose. With multi trauma, the liver injury may be the most significant or of lesser consequence than the other injuries. There may be a paucity of findings on abdominal examination, even with a significant haemoperitoneum. There may be tenderness over the lower right ribs and right upper quadrant of the abdomen and there may be some

Prof. Russell W. Strong CMG FRCS FRACS FACS FRACDS, Professor and Director of Surgery, Princess Alexandra Hospital, Ipswich Road, Woolloongabba, Queensland 4102, Australia

referred shoulder pain. Altered consciousness as a result of head injury, inebriation or the necessity to paralyse and intubate the patient, devalues the abdominal examination. Haemoglobin estimation to assess intra-abdominal bleeding will be unreliable when haemorrhage occurs from other sites such as into the thorax or from pelvic and long bone fractures.

Diagnosis and resuscitation are simultaneous events. Rapid fluid resuscitation via large bore intravenous access is required for the unstable patient. Failure to respond to therapy demands continued resuscitation on the way to the operating theatre – an easy decision in the patient with abdominal distension but more difficult in the multi trauma setting, where ongoing bleeding from other sites as the cause of instability needs to be excluded. Diagnostic peritoneal lavage will rapidly define the presence of haemoperitoneum. An increasing role for ultrasonography is emerging.[1,2] The non-invasiveness and rapidity in diagnosing haemoperitoneum may well see it replacing peritoneal lavage as the preferred method in the unstable patient. A temporary response to intravenous infusion followed by instability is an indication of continuing major bleeding and the need for immediate surgery. If the patient becomes stable with 1–2 l of fluid, definitive evaluation can be performed.

NON-OPERATIVE MANAGEMENT

Over the years it had been recognised that a large number of liver injuries had stopped bleeding at the time of operation. The development and use of computerised axial tomography (CT) allowed some precision in diagnosis together with follow-up imaging which defined the natural history of these

Table 10.1 Liver Injury Scale by the American Association for the Surgery of Trauma

Grade*		Injury description
I	Haematoma	Sub-capsular, non-expanding, < 10% surface area
	Laceration	Capsular tear, non-bleeding, < 1 cm parenchymal depth
II	Haematoma	Subcapsular, non-expanding, 10–50% surface area; intraparenchymal, non-expanding, < 2 cm in diameter
	Laceration	Capsular tear, active bleeding: 1–3 cm parenchymal depth, 10 cm in length
III	Haematoma	Subcapsular, > 50% surface area or expanding; ruptured subcapsular haematoma with active bleeding; intraparenchymal haematoma > 2 cm or expanding
	Laceration	> 3 cm parenchymal depth
IV	Haematoma	Ruptured intraparenchymal haematoma with active bleeding
	Laceration	Parenchymal disruption involving 25–50% of hepatic lobe
V	Haematoma	Parenchymal disruption involving > 50% of hepatic lobe
	Laceration	Juxtahepatic venous injuries, i.e. retrohepatic vena cava/major hepatic veins
VI	Vascular	Hepatic avulsion

injuries. A specific policy towards non-operative treatment was instituted by some centres.[3,4] In a review of publications on non-operative management, Pachter and Hofstetter[5] outlined the criteria for selection, the most important of which was haemodynamic stability on admission to hospital or the achievement of such with a modest volume of intravenous fluid. Additional criteria were the presence of neurological integrity, the absence of peritoneal signs and need for excessive hepatic related transfusion.

Most injuries treated non-operatively are grades I–III of the liver injury scale of the American Association for the Surgery of Trauma (AAST) as outlined in Table 10.1. There have been some reports of successful non-operative management of grade IV and V injuries as measured by CT scanning. It must be understood that CT grading of hepatic injury does not necessarily coincide with the operative findings. Croce et al.[6] found a poor correlation between the two and this has been the personal experience of the author. The CT scan should include intravenous contrast. Free contrast in and around the liver is indicative of active bleeding (Fig. 10.1).[7] Hepatic arteriography will identify arterial bleeding which may be embolised. Failure to demonstrate arterial bleeding or achieve embolisation requires operative intervention. Contrast enhanced CT may delineate an area of hepatic necrosis (Fig. 10.2). This does not require

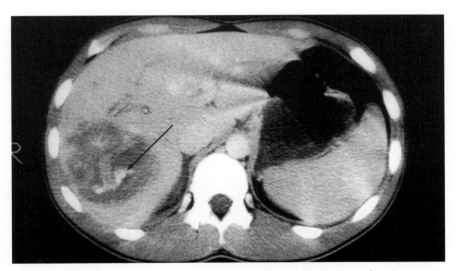

Fig. 10.1 Intravenous contrast enhanced CT scan. The arrow indicates free intravenous contrast.

Key point 1

• The most striking evolution in the management of blunt liver injuries in the past decade is the non-operative approach. This can be successful in around 80% of cases. Haemodynamic stability is the basic requirement and is supported by CT delineation of the nature and extent of the injury. Close monitoring to elucidate any change is an absolute prerequisite.

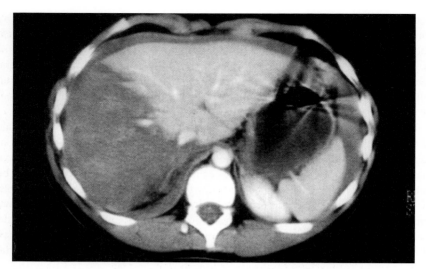

Fig. 10.2 The right hemiliver is non-perfused with intravenous contrast.

immediate intervention but planned resection is necessary. Hepatic necrosis needs to be differentiated from an intrahepatic haematoma which occupies a variable amount of space within the liver and invariably resolves (Fig. 10.3).

It is probable that 80% or more of blunt liver injuries can be successfully managed non-operatively. It requires close monitoring of vital signs, repeated examination and serial estimation of haemoglobin. While follow-up imaging to determine resolution of the injury has been advocated,[5] it has been recently advised that follow-up CT does not influence the results and is not indicated.[8] There are no rules about how long the patient needs to be rested in bed, remain in hospital or return to normal activities. Each case needs to be individually

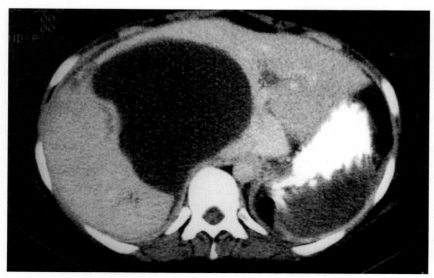

Fig. 10.3 Large intrahepatic haematoma.

treated on its merit. Early operative intervention is required if there is evidence of continuing intra-abdominal bleeding or signs of other associated injury which necessitates laparotomy. Late sequelae, such as infection of intrahepatic or subcapsular haematoma, haemobilia and major duct injury may become evident after an apparent non-complicated course and necessitate intervention. Carillo and Richardson[9] have emphasized that delayed surgery or interventional procedures should be regarded as obligatory consequences of non-operative management and not as treatment failures.

OPERATIVE MANAGEMENT

Although conservatism in the management of liver injuries has come to the fore, urgent operation is required for persistent or recurrent bleeding. This may manifest itself in three ways: (i) the shocked patient with a distended or distending abdomen; (ii) the temporary response to intravenous fluids, followed by haemodynamic instability; and (iii) on-going or recurrent bleeding following an apparent initial successful non-operative course.

Less urgent operation may be required for non-bleeding complications of the injury such as hepatic necrosis or major bile duct injury.

The surgical and anaesthetic teams must work hand-in-hand. Prolonged surgery and massive transfusion will lead to hypothermia, acidosis, coagulopathy and hypocalcaemia. Anticipation of these consequences should lead to adequate elevation of the operating theatre temperature, application of a patient warming blanket, warming devices for blood and intravenous infusions,[10] calcium infusions related to the blood transfused and correction of acidosis and coagulation defects. The successful outcome is as dependent on these parameters as it is on the surgical endeavours.

Haemorrhage is the prime indication for urgent operation and the surgeon's role is to control bleeding by whatever means. With major bleeding from a severe liver injury, the rapidity of control is a critical determinant of outcome. It takes experience and judgement to foresee the inevitable sequelae of a particular injury and to choose the appropriate course of action.[11] There are a variety of techniques that the surgeon can undertake to achieve haemostasis and the method chosen will be very dependent on the site and extent of the injury, the compounding effect of associated injuries, the general condition of the patient at the time of exploration, the expertise of the surgeon in dealing with the liver and the availability of support services. The concept of 'damage control' by an abbreviated laparotomy has evolved in the last decade[12] – do the least possible to control life-threatening injuries and come back another day. Surgical constraint should be the philosophy when faced with severe injuries, hypotension and metabolic failure. This is most likely to occur in the setting of multi trauma.

HAEMOSTATIC TECHNIQUES

Suturing

There is still an important role for suturing when individual bleeding sites are evident. Bleeding that occurs from within the liver substance without a visible vessel can be suture-ligated with a 2/0 or 0 absorbable suture. The suture is placed as a figure of eight which includes the liver tissue around the bleeding point. The ligation gently squeezes the liver tissue to avoid cutting through the soft parenchyma. When a large vessel such as an hepatic vein is bleeding, a 4/0 vascular suture should be chosen.

The 'liver suture' is a chromic catgut suture on a large curved needle. It is placed well back from the edge of the fracture and at a depth to embrace the full thickness of the wound. Whether placed as a simple suture, a figure of eight or through in one direction and 1 cm along the fracture is passed back through in the opposite direction, the edges are manually compressed together during ligation, to prevent too vigorous tension on the knot and liver tissue. Although condemned as causing liver necrosis and sepsis or allowing continued bleeding in the depth of the wound, the incidence of late complications are minimal when properly applied.[13]

Perihepatic packing

Laparotomy sponges are placed to compress the liver and wound edges together. They should not be packed into the wound as this will force the edges apart with tearing of hepatic veins and increased bleeding. Perihepatic packing may be used as: (i) a temporary measure to allow adequate resuscitation and during which period, other intra-abdominal injuries can be assessed and possibly treated; (ii) definitive treatment with multiple injuries or a complex liver injury beyond the surgeon's ability to manage; or (iii) an adjunct to other surgical treatment on the liver, particularly when hypothermia and coagulopathy promotes diffuse bleeding which is not possible to alleviate by other means.

While packing was used extensively for definitive control during World War II, the mortality from sepsis related to retention of packs for a week or more, caused it to be abandoned and censured. Its re-emergence as a modality of definitive haemorrhage control in a severe liver injury has been one of the most significant factors in the reduction of mortality.[14] The packs are removed when the patient is haemodynamically stable and coagulopathy is corrected –usually within 24–36 h.

Resection

Non-anatomical resection removes the injured portion of liver that is peripheral to the fracture line. It is a completion hepatectomy, the majority of which as been performed by the traumatic insult. The removal of this partially detached liver leaves one surface for haemorrhage control. Anatomical resection is performed along formal anatomical planes that are unrelated to the fracture lines – right and left hemihepatectomy; left lateral segment resection; segmental resection. It achieves the dual roles of removal of the source of bleeding and the site of necrosis.

Anatomical resection for trauma was once advocated but the high mortality rate caused most authorities over the past decade to condemn the procedure. Certainly many patients underwent major resections that would be regarded as unnecessary and inappropriate today. There have continued to be proponents of anatomical resection for severe liver injuries although they are a minority group and usually specialist hepatobiliary surgeons.[15–18] It is probable that should anatomical resection be required, the highest order of competence in resective liver surgery is essential and the novice should not embark on a learning curve. Resection may be required at the original operation as the only method to salvage a patient from exsanguination or in a patient where haemorrhage has been controlled by other methods but the liver is so badly damaged that it is unlikely to function normally and necrosis and sepsis will jeopardise survival.

Additional methods

Absorbable mesh compression wrap has been advocated,[19] but appears to have a limited place. When surface ooze occurs from decapsulated liver, the argon beam coagulator followed by fibrin glue and a sheet of Surgicel (Ethicon, Somerville, NJ, USA) may be beneficial. Hepatic artery ligation is rarely useful in blunt trauma where the major source of bleeding is venous. Selective hepatic arteriography and embolisation does have a place in the treatment of the rare arterio-venous fistula or haemobilia.

OPERATIVE STRATEGIES

Abdominal exploration is performed through a midline incision. Following evacuation of the haemoperitoneum, a rapid laparotomy is made to assess intra-abdominal injuries. The surgeon should not be distracted by minor injuries or sites of bleeding, but should concentrate on immediate control of major haemorrhage and thereby allow the restoration of blood volume by the anaesthetist. An unsuspected liver injury may be discovered during laparotomy for abdominal trauma. If the injury is not bleeding – do not start it! Exploring the fracture must be resisted. If the liver is bleeding, compress the fracture closed. If bleeding is curtailed, maintain compression for 20 min by the clock. If haemostasis is achieved, the fracture should not be opened as recurrent haemorrhage will ensue.

When compression fails to stop bleeding, inflow occlusion should be applied by using a flat non-crushing bowel clamp across the hepato-duodenal ligament. If bleeding is controlled, intermittent release will identify bleeding sites which can be suture-ligated. When inflow occlusion fails to control haemorrhage, hepatic venous bleeding is the cause. While maintaining inflow occlusion combined with adequate suction and vision, bleeding sites can be suture-ligated. When controlled, intermittent release of the inflow occlusion will allow bleeding hepatic artery and portal vein sites to be identified and controlled by suture ligation.

Direct haemostasis by the above methods requires a good view into the depths of the injury. The majority of blunt liver injuries involve the middle of the right hemiliver, with extension of fractures across the dome to the posterior aspect. The liver is positioned high under the costal margin which inhibits easy access. A right transverse subcostal extension from the midline incision, combined with a suitable retractor fixed to the operating table improves the exposure. Despite this manoeuvre, there is an inadequate view of many right sided injuries and complete mobilisation of the right hemiliver is necessary. This may be a daunting prospect for surgeons who are unaccustomed to dealing with the liver. It may be elected to insert 'liver sutures' without mobilising the liver. Control of haemorrhage by packing may be the most expeditious and sensible procedure for most surgeons. If this controls

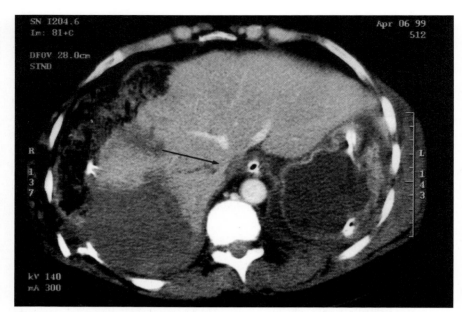

Fig. 10.4 Liver injury that has been packed - arrow shows a severely compressed inferior vena cava.

haemorrhage, do no more. Close the abdomen and transfer the patient to the intensive care unit. If packing controls major haemorrhage but there is still some bleeding which can be comfortably replaced, accept this and call for help from a surgeon who is experienced in liver surgery. Unstable patients do badly when transported and it may well be appropriate for an experienced liver surgeon to travel to the referring institution to control the situation.

Perihepatic packing should exert enough compression to control haemor-rhage but no more than is necessary. Marked compression of the IVC may partially or completely obstruct venous return which will have consequences on haemodynamic parameters, renal function and cause lower body oedema. Excessive packing could compromise respiratory function by direct pressure on the diaphragm together with increased intra-abdominal pressure from intestinal oedema which is secondary to portal venous outflow obstruction, fluid resuscitation and prolonged prolapse of bowel outside the abdomen. Although it has been stated that packing should not be so forceful as to cause an abdominal compartment syndrome,[20] if this is the only way to obtain haemostasis, it is acceptable in the short-term (Fig. 10.4). The author has experience of four cases where IVC obstruction was caused by the surgeon needing to pack with great force to obtain haemostasis and they are alive following urgent resection within 6–12 h.

There are occasions when packing fails to alleviate bleeding but does so when combined with inflow occlusion. Alternatively, some patients have the bleeding controlled by packing but become unstable after abdominal closure. Re-operation reveals haemorrhage which is controlled by inflow occlusion. The cause is hepatic vein outflow obstruction, either from the pressure exerted by the packing or the major hepatic vein being transected or sutured. Selective inflow occlusion will resolve the problem and may be accomplished by: (i)

Key point 2

- For simple liver injuries, bimanual compression, suture ligation or appropriate placement of liver sutures may suffice. The use of inflow occlusion may facilitate these steps. When faced with major haemorrhage from a severe liver injury, the concept of surgical constraint and 'damage control' has come to the fore. Therapeutic packing should be performed early and not as a last resort when all else has failed. Perihepatic packing has evolved as the most significant therapeutic modality in the reduction of mortality after a severe liver injury. Completion, non-anatomical resection has a place, whereas anatomic resection, when required, probably needs the involvement of an experienced liver surgeon.

extra hepatic control of the right hepatic artery and right portal vein; (ii) mass control of the right portal triad by the posterior Glissonian approach;[21] and (iii) placing a large suture (Fig. 10.5) which is a quick method of encompassing the right portal structures.

To rapidly perform the first two methods may be outside the scope of many general surgeons, whereas the third method can be relatively easily applied. If selective right inflow occlusion is performed, then subsequent right hemihepatectomy will be required but this can be delayed until the patient is stable – a form of 'damage control'.

While there are some liver injuries that are beyond surgical resurrection, most are treatable but the patient may be non-salvageable because of time delay from injury to operation or a cycle of events where attempts at haemostasis have resulted in hypotension, restitution of blood volume, further bleeding and hypotension, acidosis, hypothermia, etc.[22,23] The surgeon-controlled factors of

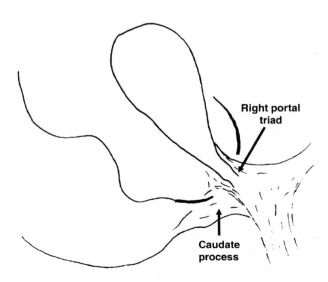

Fig. 10.5 Placement of a large suture to rapidly encompass the right portal triad.

rapid transfer to the operating theatre and expeditious control of major haemorrhage are of paramount importance. Therefore, when faced with a severe liver injury, forget the niceties of a visually pleasing repair and concentrate on saving the patient's life. The patient who has not died from exsanguination has the potential to undergo appropriate liver surgery under more controlled conditions, during a staged re-operation.

When massive oedema of the gastrointestinal tract and retroperitoneum occur, abdominal wall closure is not possible. The insertion of a silastic mesh or waterproof plastic barrier will allow the abdominal contents to be retained without excessive intra-abdominal pressure and its sequelae on respiratory and renal function.[12]

SUBCAPSULAR HAEMATOMA

A small subcapsular haematoma that is found at operation can be left alone. Likewise, a subcapsular haematoma detected on CT scan, with no compression or liver deplacement, can usually be observed. In contradistinction, an expanding or large haematoma which is compressing the liver, indicates high pressure arterial bleeding from a deeper parenchymal disruption. Continued high pressure bleeding will strip the capsule until such time as it ruptures or completely denudes the lobe. The large surface area of oozing liver is difficult to control, even with the argon beam coagulator, fibrin glue and Surgicel, with or without packing. Hepatic arteriography to identify and embolise the visible bleeding site can be attempted. The author has found surgery to be the most satisfactory treatment, with evacuation of the haematoma together with appropriate management of the disrupted parenchyma and bleeding artery.

COAGULOPATHY

Major liver trauma is frequently associated with coagulopathy.[24,25] The dilutional effect of massive transfusion on platelets and clotting factors and the adverse effects of acidosis and hypothermia are prominent.[26] The liver plays an important role in haemostasis. Procoagulant, anticoagulant and fibrinolytic proteins are synthesised in the liver[27] and injury to the liver, combined with ischaemia from hypotension, inflow occlusion, handling and compression will have deleterious effects on these haemostatic functions. These problems need to be anticipated, with steps taken to prevent or minimise them where possible by warming the theatre, the patient, the intravenous infusion and correcting acidosis and prophylactically replacing blood components. Despite these efforts, diffuse oozing from the liver and other exposed surfaces may occur. Endeavours at surgical control will fail and packing to produce tamponade will be necessary.

POSTOPERATIVE CARE

Positive pressure ventilation should be maintained until pulmonary function is restored and after any planned re-operation and will need to be prolonged when there is major thoracic trauma. Rewarming the patient and correction of coagulopathy and acidosis are essential. The failure of drains to adequately allow the egress of blood and clots means that, when present, they are unreliable as a measure of blood loss. Identification of re-bleeding is made by close monitoring of vital signs, increasing abdominal distension and a falling haemoglobin.

When perihepatic packs have been inserted, re-operation is performed at the most expeditious time after the patient is stable, normothermic and the best correction of any coagulopathy has been obtained. The operation should be undertaken by an experienced surgeon who is able to cope with the wide spectrum of procedures that may be required. This may necessitate transfer of a stable patient to a specialised unit. When the packs are removed, there may be no bleeding and no sign of bile leak or necrosis. On the other hand, bleeding may not recur but there is non-viable or macerated liver and resection is required at this time. If bleeding recurs following pack removal, a critical decision must be made to either repack or gain control by surgical means. This is the most appropriate time to carry out definitive surgery with a stable, non-coagulopathic patient and, therefore, the need for the procedure to be performed by an experienced liver surgeon.

Deranged liver function tests will be evident after major liver trauma and large transfusion requirements and they will be magnified if a substantial volume of liver has been removed. The level of bilirubin and transaminases will increase and a fall in albumin is to be expected. Salt-poor albumin infusions may be necessary. Following a major liver resection and during the process of hypertrophy the alkaline phosphatase and gamma-glutamyl transferase will rise before returning to normal levels.

An external biliary fistula occurs in up to 10% of patients with a blunt liver injury. Most fistulae will close within 3 weeks. If drainage continues for a longer period, a large hepatic duct disruption should be suspected and endoscopic retro-grade cholangiography performed. Depending on the findings, an endoscopic stent may encourage the fistula to close.[28] A late stricture will probably require surgical intervention. Haemobilia is a rare late complication. Hepatic arteriography and embolisation of the pseudo aneurysm is curative in most cases.

The presence of non-viable tissue with blood and bile collections will act as a nidus for infection which will be promoted by the immunosuppression that is a recognised consequence of trauma.[29] Hollow viscus perforation from the trauma will exacerbate the likelihood of a subphrenic abscess. The removal of devitalised liver at the time of surgery will reduce the chances of sepsis and multi organ failure. In the patient who shows signs of sepsis, there needs to be an aggressive search for the site of infection which is most likely to be elucidated by CT scan. When there is a fluid collection, percutaneous drainage by the radiologist is appropriate whereas particulate matter and course debris requires open surgery for eradication.

Key points for clinical practice

- .The most striking evolution in the management of blunt liver injuries in the past decade is the non-operative approach. This can be successful in around 80% of cases. Haemodynamic stability is the basic requirement and is supported by CT delineation of the nature and extent of the injury. Close monitoring to elucidate any change is an absolute prerequisite.

Key points for clinical practice (continued)

- For simple liver injuries, bimanual compression, suture ligation or appropriate placement of liver sutures may suffice. The use of inflow occlusion may facilitate these steps. When faced with major haemorrhage from a severe liver injury, the concept of surgical constraint and 'damage control' has come to the fore. Therapeutic packing should be performed early and not as a last resort when all else has failed. Perihepatic packing has evolved as the most significant therapeutic modality in the reduction of mortality after a severe liver injury. Completion, non-anatomical resection has a place, whereas anatomic resection, when required, probably needs the involvement of an experienced liver surgeon.

References

1. Rozycki GS, Shackford SR. Ultrasound, what every trauma surgeon should know. J Trauma 1996; 40: 1–4.
2. McGahan JP, Richards JR. Blunt abdominal trauma: the role of emergent sonography and review of the literature. Am J Roentgenol 1999; 172: 897–903.
3. Knudson MM, Lim RC, Oakes DD, Jeffery RB. Non-operative management of blunt liver injuries: the need for continued surveillance. J Trauma 1990; 30: 1494–1500.
4. Carillo EH, Platz A, Miller FB, Richardson JD, Polk HC. Non-operative management of blunt hepatic trauma. Br J Surg 1998; 85: 461–468.
5. Pachter HL, Hofstetter SR. The current status of non-operative management of adult hepatic injuries. Am J Surg 1995; 169: 442–454.
6. Croce MA, Fabian TC, Kudsk KA et al. AAST organ injury scale: correlation of CT-graded liver injuries and operative findings. J Trauma 1991; 31: 806–812.
7. Fang JF, Chen RJ, Wong YC et al. Pooling of contrast material on computed tomography mandates aggressive management of blunt hepatic trauma. Am J Surg 1998; 14: 483–486.
8. Davis KA, Brody JM, Cioffi WG. Computed tomography in blunt hepatic trauma. Arch Surg 1996; 131: 255–260.
9. Carillo EH, Richardson JD. Delayed surgery and interventional procedures in complex liver injuries. J Trauma. 1999; 46: 978.
10. Hirshberg A, Sheffer N, Barnea O. Computer simulation of hypothermia during 'damage control' laparotomy. World J Surg 1999; 23: 960–965.
11. Garrison JR, Richardson JD, Hilakos G et al. Predicting the need to pack early for severe intra-abdominal haemorrhage. J Trauma 1996; 40: 923–929.
12. Burch JM, Ortiz VB, Richardson RJ et al. Abbreviated laparotomy and planned reoperation for critically injured patients. Ann Surg 1991; 215: 476–484.
13. Stain SC, Yellin AE, Donovan AJ. Hepatic trauma. Arch Surg 1988; 123: 123–147.
14. Pachter HL, Feliciano DV. Complex hepatic injuries. Surg Clin North Am 1996; 76: 763–782.
15. Kasai T, Kobayashi K. Searching for the best operative modality for severe hepatic injuries. Surg Gynecol Obstet 1993; 77: 551–555.
16. Menegaux F, Langlois P, Chigot JP. Severe blunt trauma of the liver: a study of mortality factors. J Trauma 1993; 35: 865–869.
17. Peitzmann AB, Udekwu AO, Iwatsuki S. Resection: optimal therapy for major liver injury. In: Summons RL, Udekwu AO. (eds) Debates in Clinical Surgery, vol I Chicago: Year Book Medical Publishers 1990; 152–161.
18. Strong RW, Lynch SV, Wall DR, Liu CL. Anatomic resection for severe liver trauma. Surgery 1998; 123: 251–257.
19. Stevens SL, Maull KI, Enderson M et al. Total mesh wrapping for parenchymal liver injuries: a combined experimental and clinical study. J Trauma 1991; 31: 1103–1108.

20. Meldrum DR, Moore FA, Moore EE et al. Cardiopulmonary hazards of perihepatic packing for major liver injuries. Am J Surg 1995; 170: 537–542.
21. Launois B, Jamieson GG. The posterior intrahepatic approach for hepatectomy or removal of segments of the liver. Surg Gynecol Obstet 1992; 174: 155–158.
22. Beal SL. Fatal hepatic haemorrhage: an unresolved problem in the management of complex liver injuries. J Trauma 1990; 30: 163–169.
23. Hirshberg A, Wall MJ, Mattox KL. Planned re-operation for trauma: a two year experience with 124 consecutive patients. J Trauma 1994; 37: 365–369.
24. Harrigan C, Lucas CE, Ledgerwood AM. The effects of haemorrhagic shock on the clotting cascade in injured patients. J Trauma 1989; 29: 1416–1422.
25. Wudel JH, Morris JA, Yates K et al. Massive transfusion: outcome in blunt trauma patients. J Trauma 1991; 31: 1–7.
26. Cosgriff N, Moore EE, Sauaia A et al. Predicting life-threatening coagulopathy in the massively transfused trauma patient: hypothermia and acidosis revisited. J Trauma 1997; 42: 857–862.
27. Castelino DJ, Salem HH. Natural anticoagulants and the liver. J Gastroenterol Hepatol 1997; 12: 77–83.
28. Krige JE, Bornman PC, Terblanche J. Liver trauma in 446 patients. S Afr J Surg 1997; 35: 10–15.
29. Moore FA, Moore EE. Evolving concepts in the pathogenesis of post-injury organ failure. Surg Clin North Am 1995; 75: 257–277.

The management of blunt liver injuries

D.J. Gouma   H. Obertop

Operative bile duct injury

Since its introduction in the late 1980s, laparoscopic cholecystectomy has been generally accepted as the treatment of choice for symptomatic gallstone disease and has replaced the conventional 'open' cholecystectomy. More than 75% of cholecystectomies are now performed laparoscopically.[1]

Several studies have shown the efficacy and safety of the procedure as well as the advantages such as reduced hospital stay, earlier recovery, less intra-abdominal adhesions and a better cosmetic outcome.[2] Laparoscopic cholecystectomy can also be performed safely as a day-care procedure.[3]

Unfortunately, this minimally invasive technique is associated with a higher incidence of bile duct injury (BDI).[4–6] However, the incidence of BDI is strongly related to experience and recently a decrease in BDI has been reported.[7–9]

Despite knowledge on the mechanism of injury and many reports which stress the value of preventive measures such as intra-operative cholangiography, the reported incidence still varies between 0–1%.[5,6,10] Bile duct injuries after laparoscopic cholecystectomy are frequently seen in HPB surgery referral centres.[11]

Early diagnosis and classification of the severity of BDI and careful selection of the different treatment modalities, in particular selection for the endoscopic or surgical approach is crucial for successful outcome.

Inadequate management of BDI may lead to severe complications, such as biliary peritonitis leading to sepsis and multiple organ failure in the early phase, and biliary cirrhosis during long-term follow-up, eventually leading to the need for liver transplantation.

Since the introduction of laparoscopic cholecystectomy, around 200 patients with BDI have been treated at the Amsterdam Academic Medical Center (AMC), a referral centre for HPB surgery. The management of these patients is

Professor Dr D.J. Gouma, Department of Surgery, Academic Medical Center, G4-116, Meibergdreef 9, 1105 AZ Amsterdam, The Netherlands (for correspondence)
Professor Dr H. Obertop, Department of Surgery, Academic Medical Center, G4-116, Meibergdreef 9, 1105 AZ Amsterdam, The Netherlands

> ## Key point 1
>
> • Diagnostic work-up and treatment of bile duct injuries needs a multidisciplinary approach (gastroenterologists, radiologists, surgeons).

always discussed in a multidisciplinary team consisting of gastroenterologists, radiologists and surgeons.

This review summaries the management of these patients and discusses the incidence, symptoms, classification of the severity of the injury and, in particular, the surgical treatment.

INCIDENCE OF BILIARY INJURY IN OPEN AND LAPAROSCOPIC CHOLECYSTECTOMY

The incidence of BDI after cholecystectomy varies widely and is reported between 0 and more than 1% in several studies, a difference that is partly due to the various definitions of bile duct injury.[1,2,4–11] In some series, leakage of a cystic duct or duct of Luschka is also included as an injury (minor injuries) whereas in other studies only the more severe common bile duct injuries such as transection and resection are included and reported as major injuries.[5,6] The incidence in the different studies is also influenced by the selection of patients as well as the methods for data collection (audit versus interview).[1,2,5,7–9]

In two reviews, the incidence after an open procedure was reported as 0.2% (McMahon) and 0.7% (Strasberg) whereas the incidence after laparoscopic cholecystectomy was, respectively, 0.81% and 0.5%.[5,6] In a survey from The Netherlands shortly after the introduction of laparoscopic cholecystectomy in 1991, the incidence was 0.86%.[4] Limited experience correlated significantly with an increasing probability of a bile duct injury.[7]

In a recent audit from the west of Scotland of nearly 6000 patients, the incidence of BDI after laparoscopic cholecystectomy decreased from 0.8% in 1990–1993 to 0.4% during 1995.[8]

Nair et al.[9] recently reported a survey from England with an incidence of 0.07% in 4000 patients. An underestimation of the real incidence of BDI in this study is probable because the incidence is lower than in any other non-selected 'nation-wide' series.[1,4,5,6,10]

Around 11,000 laparoscopic cholecystectomies are performed in The Netherlands each year and this should result in about 30 BDI incidents according to the recent suggestions of lower incidence of injuries. The number of patients referred to the AMC (one of the eight university hospitals) has not decreased during the past years and is currently at 30–35 patients per year.[12] This does not provide conclusions about the incidence of BDI but may reflect a change in referral pattern.

CLASSIFICATION

The generally accepted Bismuth classification for bile duct lesions relates to the level of injury but not to the nature of the lesion and, therefore, can not be used for all injuries, especially not bile leaks after laparoscopic surgery.[13] New classification systems for a bile duct injury have been developed during the past years. McMahon et al.[5] suggested a division into major and minor bile duct injuries. Strasberg et al.[6] reported a very detailed classification (type A to E) including many subclassifications (E1 to E4). In 1993, we introduced a relatively simple classification with direct implications for further treatment.[14]

In this classification, a bile duct injury is defined as any clinically evident damage to the biliary system including the cystic duct and intrahepatic duct radicals. Four types of bile duct injury can be identified:

A. Cystic duct leaks or leakage from aberrant or peripheral hepatic radicles including the so-called duct of Luschka.

B. Major bile duct leaks with or without concomitant biliary strictures.

C. Bile duct strictures without bile leakage.

D. Complete transection of the bile duct with or without excision of a part of the bile duct.

It was found that both treatment and prognosis of a bile duct injury are mainly dependent on the nature of the lesion according to this classification as will be discussed below. Therefore, this classification is helpful in evaluating results of BDI treatment.

DIAGNOSIS

CLINICAL PRESENTATION

The time interval between laparoscopic cholecystectomy and the detection of the lesion varies widely and three different groups of patients with bile duct injury can be identified. They have different clinical symptoms and should be investigated and treated differently.

The injury is detected during laparoscopic cholecystectomy
In a nation-wide study from The Netherlands about one-third of lesions were detected during the initial surgical procedure which is in accordance with the literature.[4] Detection of an injury during the procedure was not dependent on the use of routine peri-operative cholangiography. It has been suggested that the majority of injuries will be detected during the procedure. There are no data available to support this suggestion.

Only 16% of the injuries referred to the AMC were detected during the procedure and this has not changed throughout the years. This may be due to the selection of patients referred.[11,14]

Most patients with a diagnosis at the time of operation are treated immediately, generally after conversion to an open procedure and referral of these patients is thereby very selected. Generally, only patients with extensive injuries (Fig. 11.1) or failures after primary repair at the initial procedure are referred.

Patients with delayed identification (> 24 h after surgery) of a bile duct injury
These patients are diagnosed postoperatively after a median interval of 7 days.[11] In our series, symptoms in the early postoperative phase were non-

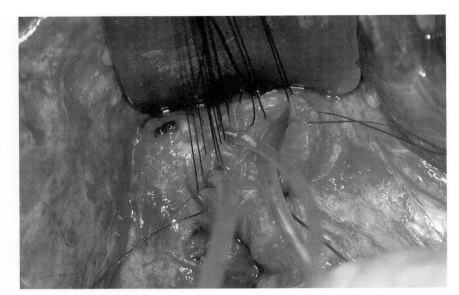

Fig. 11.1 A patient with a bile duct injury detected during laparoscopic cholecystectomy. After conversion to an open procedure extension of the injury into 4 segmental intrahepatic ducts occurred. Sutures are placed at the proximal border of the bile ducts and the ducts are stented by catheters. The ducts were connected and a double hepaticojejunostomy was performed.

specific and consisted of general malaise, nausea, vomiting, anorexia, abdominal pain and low grade fever. The non-specificity of these symptoms is probably responsible for the delay in diagnosis. These patients were frequently discharged from hospital on the second postoperative day and re-admitted after a few days because of persistent complaints. Other symptoms may become manifest later and consist of sepsis and jaundice and in most patients the symptoms eventually lead to the (delayed) detection of the injury.

Patients with delayed detection of injuries can be divided into two subgroups: (i) patients with biliary leakage immediately or a few days after laparoscopic cholecystectomy resulting in a biloma and biliary peritonitis: or (ii) patients with total occlusion (clipping) of the common bile duct leading to early obstructive jaundice frequently followed after 1–2 weeks by biliary leakage and biliary peritonitis due to the increasing intraductal pressure and subsequent leakage at the site of the clips.

The presenting symptoms may vary widely and are frequently not in accordance with the severity of the injury or extent of the intra-abdominal fluid/bile collection. A biloma can exist for a long period of time before symptoms occur. Therefore, symptoms are generally not a guide to treatment strategy except for urgent laparotomy due to persistent severe biliary peritonitis with sepsis.

In patients analyzed in the period after introduction of laparoscopic cholecystectomy (1990–1994), symptoms occurred 3–5 days after the procedure and a bile duct injury was detected after a mean period of 9 days after the first symptoms (latency time). In a later period (1995–1996) the latency time between symptoms and diagnosis decreased significantly from 9 days to 3.5 days (P <0.05).[11] There is more awareness of the possibility of BDI after laparoscopic cholecystectomy than in previous years.

Patients with a relatively long symptom-free interval (even greater than 1 year).

These patients present with obstructive jaundice due to a stricture frequently without cholangitis (Fig. 11.2). It has been suggested that these late bile duct strictures originate mainly from ischaemic lesions caused by extensive dissection, or partial occlusion of the common duct with a clip during the initial procedure.

DIAGNOSTIC PROCEDURES

An early diagnosis is important and can easily be established by ultrasound which is helpful in the detection of a fluid collection and bile duct dilatation. Subsequent percutaneous aspiration of bile will establish the diagnosis. A fluid collection (suggesting a bile duct lesion) is still an indication for exploratory laparotomy for many surgeons leading to unnecessary surgery for bile drainage which might lead to unnecessary exploration of the bile duct. Laparotomy should be avoided at this stage. In our series, about 30% of the patients were referred after one or more 'diagnostic' and unnecessary explorative laparotomies.[11]

Key point 2

- 'Diagnostic' laparotomy should be avoided in patients suspected having a bile duct injury.

The next step is visualization of the biliary tract by magnetic resonance cholangio-pancreatography (MRCP) or ERCP not only to establish the diagnosis, but to identify the nature and level of the lesion (Figs 11.2 & 11.3A,B).

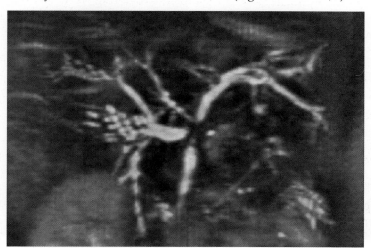

Fig. 11.2 A patient with obstructive jaundice 6 months after laparoscopic cholecystectomy. A clip was removed 2 days after the initial procedure without further complications, but cholangitis occurred after 6 months. MRCP showed a hilar stricture into the segmental intrahepatic ducts.

Key point 3

- Visualization of the biliary tract by MRCP, ERCP or PTC is not only indicated to establish the diagnosis but to identify the nature and extent of the lesion.

If MRCP is not available and ERCP only shows the distal bile duct occluded with a clip, a percutaneous transhepatic pancreatography (PTC) can be performed to visualize the proximal biliary tract. Subsequent percutaneous biliary drainage can be performed (Fig. 11.3A,B).

When an abdominal drain is still in situ, cholangiography can be performed by this route (drainography; Fig. 11.4A,B).

Surgical reconstruction without visualization of the entire biliary system should not be attempted.

TREATMENT

In this review only the surgical treatment will be discussed in detail. The multidisciplinary approach (gastroenterologists, radiologists, surgeons) is, however, advocated not only for the diagnostic work-up but also to select patients for different treatment modalities. The important role of non-surgical treatment has previously been reported.[11,12,14,15] One should realize that not all forms of treatment are available in every hospital. Therefore, treatment

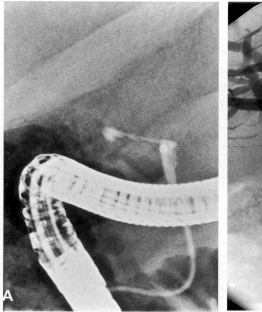
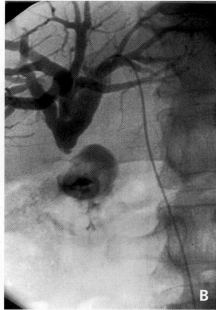

Fig. 11.3 An ERCP in a patient with a stricture of the CBD and leakage (**A**). A subsequent PTC showed a stenosis at the hilum with bile leakage and a spontaneous fistula to the transverse colon (**B**). Elective repair by hepaticojejunostomy was performed after 8 weeks of biliary drainage.

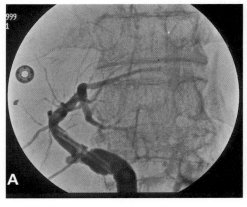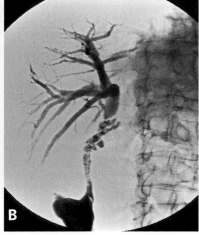

Fig. 11.4 A patient with persistent biliary leakage from an abdominal drain after cholecystectomy. Cholangiography did not show any leakage (**A**) and was considered to be normal. A subsequent X-ray through the drain showed leakage of the right hepatic duct (**B**). A hepaticojejunostomy on the right hepatic duct was performed.

principles as outlined below are only useful and applicable in centres with sufficient experience in interventional radiology, therapeutic endoscopy and reconstructive surgery.

Inadequate diagnostic work-up and subsequent suboptimal treatment of these injuries is not acceptable nowadays,[16,17] as many experienced centres report excellent results of repair procedures.[14,18–21]

Treatment of injuries detected during laparoscopic cholecystectomy

If a bile duct injury is detected during laparoscopic cholecystectomy, one should consult a surgeon with sufficient experience in hepatobiliary surgery. This experience is important as extension of the injuries into the intrahepatic ducts (Fig. 11.1) or subsequent damage to the arterial supply (bleeding and clipping or ligation of right hepatic artery) can occur.

With the help of an experienced HPB surgeon, further laparoscopic or open exploration can be performed to identify the structures in the hepatoduodenal ligament and the severity of the injury. If the local anatomy is still unclear, one should abandon further exploration and perform adequate drainage only. Direct cholangiography with catheters into the open ductal system may be helpful to identify the extent of the lesion.

If a common bile duct lesion is adequately identified and not associated with extensive damage or tissue loss and thus suitable for primary repair, an end-to-end anastomosis should be performed over a T-tube for drainage. This procedure is associated with a high incidence of late bile duct strictures, but provides optimal internal biliary drainage with a reasonable chance for cure. It also creates the optimal circumstances for reconstructive surgery by means of an elective hepatojejunostomy at a later stage.

Even endoscopic stenting and/or balloon dilatation may be successful in these patients after primary repair and even if not successful does not adversely effect surgical reconstruction.[12,15,22]

Later reconstructive surgery by elective hepatojejunostomy for stenosis of an end-to-end anastomosis has a higher success rate that acute reconstruction with a hepatojejunostomy on a non-dilated bile duct.

If part of the bile duct is accidentally resected but the proximal duct is well below the bifurcation of the hepatic duct and local circumstances (experience) are optimal, an acute reconstruction by a hepatojejunostomy can be performed. For higher lesions at the bifurcation or intrahepatically located, without a dilated ductal system adequate drainage is indicated and patients should be referred for elective reconstruction.

If local experience is limited at the time of detection of the injury, one should only perform a drainage procedure and refer the patient to an experienced centre. Simple drainage of the right upper abdomen and referral to a centre has not been shown to have a negative effect on outcome.

Key point 4

- Simple drainage of the right upper abdomen and referral to a centre has not been shown to have a negative effect on outcome and should be preferred if experience is limited.

Treatment of injuries detected later

Patients with bile duct injuries, detected at a later phase should never undergo exploration before classification of the injury, except in patients with severe biliary peritonitis who cannot be managed by percutaneous drainage. In

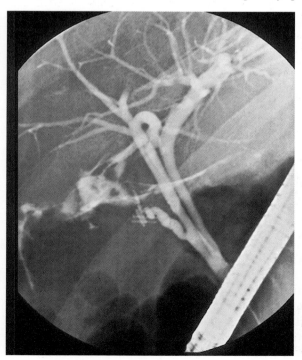

Fig. 11.5 A cystic stump leakage (type A) detected 5 days after laparoscopic cholecystectomy demonstrated by ERCP and treated by endoscopic sphincterotomy and stent for 6 weeks. Note the low bifurcation of the right and left hepatic duct.

patients with delayed diagnosis, drainage should be performed preferably by ERCP and stent insertion or PTC (Fig. 11.5). Both techniques can be combined with US or CT guided percutaneous drainage of a bile collection.[14,18,19]

An important factor for surgical outcome is the timing of reconstruction. It has been suggested that surgical reconstruction by hepatojejunostomy in the 'late' acute postoperative phase (often in a patient with bile leakage and subsequent peritonitis, ileus and the presence of local inflammatory changes in the hepatoduodenal ligament) is associated with a higher risk of postoperative complications such as bile leakage and eventually stenosis of the anastomosis. Therefore, patients are sent home with a drainage catheter and collection bag and some of these patients will have a nasogastric tube or a percutaneous gastric catheter to replace bile into the duodenum. When an exploration is performed for drainage of a bile collection after unsuccessful attempt at repair, a small bore feeding jejunostomy can be performed to enable re-insertion of bile into the GI tract. Reconstruction of the biliary tract is performed electively after 6–8 weeks. During exploration, there is generally a (dense) inflammatory reaction and fibrosis around the area of injury.

Exploration is started by mobilization of the transverse colon and duodenum from the liver, and in particular the gallbladder bed. The hepatoduodenal ligament is dissected next and the hepatic artery can always be identified as a marker as well as the portal vein. In some patients, however, local fibrosis makes dissection of the portal vein difficult. Therefore, dissecting towards the liver hilum and early lowering of the hepatic duct remnant by dividing the hilar plate as described by Couinaud and Bismuth and recommended by Blumgart is mandatory to minimize dissection between the duct remnant and portal vein.[23] The percutaneous drain, the drain tract or PTC catheter can be used as a guidance in the hilum to the damaged duct.

After puncture and opening of the proximal duct remnant, stay sutures are placed at the proximal border of the duct and the duct stump or different segmental bile duct stumps are further mobilized from the portal vein and the incision in the duct is enlarged. Multiple intrahepatic segmental duct stumps are mobilized and if possible sutured together before one or two jejunal anastomoses are performed. Usually normal duct mucosa can be seen after resection of the fibrotic tissue. Temporary stenting of the anastomosis is only performed in non-dilated ducts or when a percutaneous transhepatic drainage catheter is already in situ.

OUTCOME OF TREATMENT

Results from specialized centres, as recently summarized in an analysis of 40 US series, has show favourable short-term outcome.[10] However, long-term follow-up (more than 5 years) for repairs of BDI after laparoscopic chole-cystectomy are scanty.

Recently, we performed a long-term follow-up on the first 106 patients treated between 1990–1996. Results after endoscopic treatment (mainly type A and B lesions) were excellent with a 94% success rate (no recurrent symptoms, no abnormal liver function tests after 5 year).

The outcome of surgical reconstruction mainly for type C and D lesions or failure of endoscopic treatment was dependent on the timing of reconstruction. The overall success rate was 84%. In patients who underwent delayed reconstruction, 94% obtained successful results.

Patients developing a stenosis after surgical reconstruction should preferably be treated by percutaneous transhepatic pneumodilatation with a 70% long-term success rate. In some patients, secondary percutaneous dilatation can be successfully performed.[24]

CONCLUSIONS

The incidence of bile duct injury seems to be marginally higher after laparoscopic cholecystectomy than after open surgery. A decrease in the incidence of injuries has been reported recently. Management in terms of early diagnosis and classification of injuries before explorative laparotomy is still suboptimal. Of patients with a bile duct injury, 30% undergo a 'diagnostic laparotomy'. Most type A and B injuries (90%) can be treated endoscopically and all type D lesions must be treated by surgical reconstruction. A delayed elective reconstruction is associated with less complications compared to acute repair under suboptimal circumstances and has a success rate of 90% in experienced centres. Simple drainage of the right upper abdomen in acute circumstances with subsequent referral to a centre does not have a negative effect on outcome.

Key points for clinical practice

- Diagnostic work up and treatment of bile duct injuries needs a multidisciplinary approach (gastroenterologists, radiologists, surgeons).

- 'Diagnostic' laparotomy should be avoided in patients suspected having a bile duct injury.

- Visualization of the biliary tract by ERCP, ERCP or PTC is not only indicated to establish the diagnosis but to identify the nature and extent of the lesion.

- Simple drainage of the right upper abdomen and referral to a centre has not been shown to have a negative effect on outcome and should be preferred if experience is limited.

- Surgical reconstruction for delayed detected bile duct injuries in the early postoperative phase is associated with a higher risk for complication compared with elective repair after 6–8 weeks.

References

1. Fletcher DR, Hobbs MST, Tan P et al. Complications of cholecystectomy: risks of the laparoscopic approach and protective effects of operative cholangiography. A population based study. Ann Surg 1999; 229: 449–457.
2. Deziel DJ, Millikan KW, Exonomou SG, Doolas A, Ko ST, Airan MC. Complications of laparoscopic cholecystectomy: a national survey of 4,292 hospitals and an analysis of 77,604 cases. Am J Surg 1993; 165: 9–14.
3. Keulemans YCA, Eshuis J, Haes de H, Wit de LT, Gouma DJ. Laparoscopic cholecystectomy: day-care versus clinical observation. Ann Surg 1998; 228: 734–740.
4. Go PMNYH, Schol FPG, Gouma DJ. Laparoscopic cholecystectomy in The Netherlands. Br J Surg 1993; 80: 1180–1183.
5. McMahon AJ, Fullarton G, Baxter JN, O'Dwyer PJ. Bile duct injury and bile leakage in laparoscopic cholecystectomy. Br J Surg 1995; 82: 307–313.
6. Strasberg SM, Hertl M, Soper NJ. An analysis of the problem of biliary injury during laparoscopic cholecystectomy. J Am Coll Surg 1995; 180: 101–125.
7. Schol FPG, Go PMNYH, Gouma DJ. Risk factors for bile duct injury in laparoscopic cholecystectomy: analysis of 49 cases. Br J Surg 1994; 81: 1786–1788.
8. Richardson MC, Bell G, Fullarton GM and the West of Scotland Laparoscopic Cholecystectomy Audit Group. Incidence and nature of bile duct injuries following laparoscopic cholecystectomy: an audit of 5913 cases. Br J Surg 1996; 83: 1356–1360.
9. Nair RG, Dunn DC, Fowler S, McCloy RF. Progress with cholecystectomy: improving results in England and Wales. Br J Surg 1997; 84: 1396–1398.
10. MacFayden BV, Vecchio R, Ricardo AE, Mathis CR. Bile duct injury after laparoscopic cholecystectomy. The United States' experience. Surg Endosc 1998; 12: 315–321.
11. Keulemans YCA, Bergman JJGHM, Wit de LT et al. Improvement in the management of bile duct injuries? J Am Coll Surg 1998; 187: 246–254.
12. Gouma DJ, Rauws EAJ, Keulemans YCA, Bergman JJHGM, Huibregtse K, Obertop H. Galwegletsel na laparoscopische cholecystectomie. Ned Tijdschr Geneeskd 1999; 143: 606–611.
13. Bismuth H. Postoperative strictures of the bile duct. In: Blumgart LH (ed) The Biliary Tract. Edinburgh: Churchill Livingstone, 1982; 209–218.
14. Bergman JJGHM, Brink van den GR, Rauws EAJ et al. Treatment of bile duct lesions after laparoscopic cholecystectomy. Gut 1996; 38: 141–147.
15. Ponsky JL. Endoscopic approaches to common bile duct injuries. Laparosc Surg 1996; 76: 505–513.
16. Kern KA. Malpractice litigation involving laparoscopic cholecystectomy. Arch Surg 1997; 132: 392–398.
17. Carroll BJ, Birth M, Phillips EH. Common bile duct injuries during laparoscopic cholecystectomy that result in litigation. Surg Endosc 1998; 12: 310–314.
18. Moossa AR, Easter DW, Van Sonnenberg E, Casola G, D'Agostino H. Laparoscopic injuries to the bile duct. Ann Surg 1992; 215: 203–208.
19. Lillemoe KD, Martin SA, Cameron JL et al. Major bile duct injuries during laparoscopic cholecystectomy. Ann Surg 1997; 225: 459–471.
20. Mirza DF, Narsimhan KL, Ferraz Neto BH, Mayer AD, McMaster P, Buckels JAC. Bile duct injury following laparoscopic cholecystectomy: referral pattern and management. Br J Surg 1997; 84: 786–790.
21. Raute M, Podlech P, Aschke WJ, Manegold BC, Trede M, Chiri B. Management of bile duct injuries and strictures following cholecystectomy. World J Surg 1993; 17: 553–562.
22. Brugge WR, van Dam J. Pancreatic and biliary endoscopy. N Engl J Med 1999; 341: 1808–1816.
23. Blumgart LH. Hilar and intrahepatic biliary-enteric anastomosis. In: Blumgart LH. (ed) Surgery of the Liver and Biliary Tract, vol. II. Edinburgh: Churchill Livingstone, 1988; 899–913.
24. Vos PM, Beek van EJR, Smits NJ, Rauws EAJ, Gouma DJ, Reeders JWAJ. Percutaneous balloon dilatation for benign hepaticojejunostomy strictures. Abdom Imaging 2000; 25: 134–138.

N.E. Dudley

Adrenalectomy

Few surgical subspecialties will fail to highlight minimally invasive techniques amongst the significant advances which have taken place in their field over the last decade of the 20th century. Endocrine surgery is no exception with the beneficial impact most evident in the procedure of adrenalectomy. In comparison to cholecystectomy, where laparoscopic removal of the gallbladder was rapidly accepted as 'an advance' and became widely practised, endorsement of minimally invasive surgery for the removal of adrenal tumours has understandably been much slower. This simply reflects the rarity of adrenal surgical pathology and the difficulty of establishing a sustained learning curve for a new technique by individual surgeons. There has also been anxiety, amongst other factors, of ensuring good 'remote control' of the notorious right adrenal vein and of disturbing the intra-abdominal pressure in physiologically unstable patients principally with a phaeochromocytoma.

SURGICAL RESULTS

Until the 1990s, the 'gold standard' for patients requiring surgical adrenalectomy was either the posterior open approach for small non-malignant tumours or the lateral (subcostal) transabdominal/thoraco-abdominal approach for larger lesions greater than 5 cm in diameter and those with known or suspected malignancy. Results for these operations published by Lynn in the UK[1] (with

> **Key point 1**
> • Endoscopic adrenalectomy is the new 'gold' standard for 60% of patients requiring adrenalectomy.

N.E. Dudley MA FRCS FRCS(Ed), Honorary Consultant Surgeon, The John Radcliffe Hospital, Level 2, Headington, Oxford OX3 9DU, UK

particular reference to phaeochromocytoma) and Nash and colleagues in the US[2] challenged advocates of endoscopic adrenalectomy, pioneered by Gagner, in 1992,[3,4] to do better. The Indianapolis group were very specific in setting their 'benchmark', selecting a particularly favourable group of patients with primary aldosteronism due to a small cortical adenoma (Conn's tumour). They reported 40 cases operated upon over a 10 year period using the open posterior approach.[2] The mean operating time was 200 min and hospital stay 4.4 days. Of their patients, 15% had significant peri-operative morbidity, but in fact morbidity may have been even greater as other centres have reported disabling musculoskeletal symptoms identified on longer term follow-up.[5] These symptoms are thought to arise from excision of the twelfth rib and the occasional inevitable division of the subcostal nerve.

In the last five consecutive patients with Conn's tumour in the Oxford/ Sheffield laparoscopic adrenalectomy series,[6] mean operating time was 60 min quicker and hospital stay 1.4 days shorter than this 'benchmark'. Morbidity short- and long-term was zero.

Larger studies within single institutions have compared the three main surgical approaches – posterior open, anterior open and transperitoneal laparoscopic – across a broad range of adrenal pathologies. The aim has been to identify which operative approach is most appropriate and gives the best outcome for individual tumours.

LAPAROSCOPIC APPROACH

Prinz[7] concluded that 60% of surgically treatable adrenal disease could be approached laparoscopically and was ideal for cortical adenomas responsible for primary aldosteronism and Cushing's syndrome. Larger tumours greater than 8–10 cm diameter, typically bulky phaeochromocytomas, adrenocortical carcinomas and ganglioneuromas of the adrenal still favour an open transabdominal or an occasional thoraco-abdominal approach. Thompson and co-workers at the Mayo Clinic comparing posterior open and transperitoneal laparoscopic adrenalectomy drew similar conclusions.[5] Table 12.1 shows the demographics of their patients undergoing the two operations and matches as

Table 12.1 Demographics

	Posterior adrenalectomy (open post)	Laparoscopic adrenalectomy (transperitoneal)
Patients (*n*)	50	50
Women (%)	60	64
Mean age (years)	51	50
Primary aldosteronism (%)	50	48
Cushing's syndrome (%)	20	20
Phaeochromocytoma (%)	14	20
Non-functioning (%)	16	12
Right (%)	34	36
Left (%)	56	54
Bilateral (%)	10	10
Mean size (cm)	2.9	2.9
Mean body weight (kg)	83	78

Table 12.2 Results (mean values unless otherwise stated

	Posterior adrenalectomy	Laparoscopic adrenalectomy	*P* value
Operating room time (min)	127	167	0.0002
Blood transfusion (total group)	None	2 units	NS
Narcotic (morphine sulphate) equiv.	48	28	0.0002
Toradol doses	1.7	0.7	0.75
Anti-emetic doses	5.7	3.1	0.50
Hospital stay (days)	5.7	3.1	0.0001
Early complications (%)	18	6	0.25
Late complications (%)	54	0	0.0001
Return to normal (weeks)	7	3.8	0.0001
Patient satisfaction (1–10)*	7	9	0.0001
Adjusted hospital charges	$6,000	$7,000	0.05

*10 = most satisfied. Adapted from Thompson et al.[5]

carefully as possible the two groups with regard to gender, age, pathology, etc. Although this was neither a prospective nor randomized study it is claimed to be better than a straight retrospective review. Table 12.2 shows the results and looked for statistical differences between the two groups of patients rather than pairs of individuals. An element of bias does exist in so far as the authors have chosen to exclude 12% of the laparoscopic adrenalectomy patients who underwent conversion. This was justified because they were all in the early phase of the learning curve for the operation. The rate subsequently dropped to less than 5% and it was felt that the message for the series overall was not significantly altered. Although the laparoscopic approach was more expensive than the open procedure, there were clear advantages to laparoscopic adrenalectomy despite longer operating time. Specifically, the advantages were shorter hospitalization, reduced analgesic and anti-emetic medication and a faster return to normal physical activities.

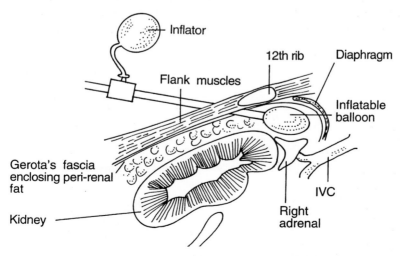

Fig. 12.1 Balloon dilator in place to create a space around the adrenal for the retroperitoneal dissection of the adrenal.

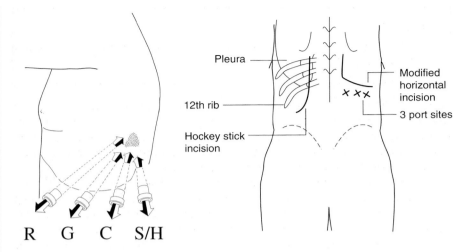

Fig. 12.2 Port sites immediately below the costal margin for standard transperitoneal laparoscopic adrenalectomy. R, retractor; G, grasping forceps; C, camera; S/H scissors/hook.

Fig. 12.3 Routine hockey stick and modified horizontal incision for open posterior adrenalectomy and port sites marked XXX for the posterior endoscopic approach.

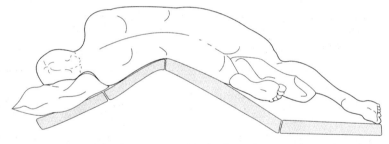

Fig. 12.4 Patient 'jack-knifed' on the table for lateral approach to adrenalectomy either by the trans- or retroperitoneal route.

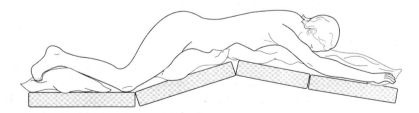

Fig. 12.5 Positioning of the patient for posterior 'open' or 'closed' adrenalectomy.

In an attempt to achieve even better results, surgeons, notably in Germany and The Netherlands, have promoted the concept of preserving the integrity of the peritoneal cavity by operating in the retroperitoneum.[8] A space within the fat around the adrenals is created by a balloon dilator directed either posteriorly with the patient jack-knifed on the table as for a traditional open posterior adrenalectomy or from the side, with the patient in the lateral decubitus position

---

Key point 2

- Transperitoneal and retroperitoneal endoscopic adrenalectomy are comparably effective.

(Figs 12.1–12.5). Duh and his colleagues[9] compared the results of 23 patients who underwent lateral laparoscopic adrenalectomy with 14 treated by the posterior endoscopic method. The patients had a variety of adrenal pathologies. The mean operating time was 3.8 h versus 3.4 h and the mean hospital stay was 2.2 days versus 1.5 days for the lateral and posterior approaches, respectively.

The conclusion reached was that in terms of patient outcomes both retroperitoneal approaches were basically the same. However, the longer operating times reflect the problem of orientation with few anatomical landmarks and the difficulty of working within a confined space. Perhaps the maximum benefit rests with the patient requiring bilateral adrenalectomy where the posterior endoscopic approach avoids time consuming and awkward repositioning of the patient. As with open posterior adrenalectomy, however, patients with larger tumours are unsuitable.

Key point 3

- Patients requiring bilateral adrenalectomy for 'end' stage Cushing's syndrome/disease remain surgically challenging whichever approach is used.

A still unresolved question is which operative approach to select for some of the most difficult patients – those with end stage Cushing's disease who have failed medical control and have not been cured by pituitary microsurgery. Obesity and extreme fragility of the tissues presents a serious challenge for whichever surgical approach is used. These patients, however, have most to benefit from endoscopic surgery which avoids large skin and muscle cutting incisions.

LOCALIZATION TECHNIQUES

All the foregoing methods of adrenalectomy rely heavily upon accurate localization of the pathological process. In the past there was no reliable alternative to formal laparotomy checking both adrenals to identify the site of the lesion and to exclude bilateral and ectopic disease. Now second generation CT, MRI, isotope scintigraphy and selective venous sampling provide localization of the surgical target with great precision as well as valuable information about anatomical relationships. Cortical adenomas as small as 2–3 mm can be identified on MRI offering the opportunity of partial adrenalectomy with preservation of the rest of the gland.

The downside of such sensitivity is that, with the ever-increasing routine use of ultrasound and CT scanning in the assessment of abdominal symptoms, many totally unsuspected adrenal tumours are now being identified. These incidentalomas are found on approximately 0.6% of all abdominal CT scans performed for unrelated conditions and their management is now becoming more standardized. All need to be investigated for adrenal hormonal over-production regardless of size. This can be achieved with speed and cost efficiency by measuring the serum potassium (aldosteronism), urinary metanephrines (phaeochromocytoma) and 24-h urinary free cortisol (hypercorticalism).

NON-FUNCTIONING TUMOURS

Adrenalectomy is fully justified if hormonal excess is identified. The management of non-functioning incidentalomas is much more problematic and controversial. The concern arises that the incidenaloma may represent a carcinoma or adrenal metastasis. In a report of 63 incidentalomas, only one was found to be functional and one malignant.[10] The latter was an adrenocortical carcinoma with a diameter of 7.0 cm. Thirty-two patients with tumours smaller than 3 cm in diameter were followed up for a mean of 18 months and only a single patient demonstrated an increase in tumour size. Adrenalectomy subsequently revealed a benign cortical adenoma. The authors suggest that all non-functioning incidentalomas larger than 3 cm should be excised.

A more liberal approach has been advocated by an Australian team justifying 60 operations for incidentalomas ± hypertension on the basis that laparoscopic adrenalectomy is quick and safe.[11] Changing the criteria for surgical intervention on the basis of technology is hard to justify and it is preferable to look for more sophisticated methods of differentiating between benign and malignant lesions. In-phase–out-of-phase MRI is highly sensitive in detecting lipid content which is rich in benign adrenal tumours but absent in metastases. The use of the corticotrophin releasing hormone test[12] or scintigraphy using [^{131}I]-6-iodomethyl norcholesterol[13] is also helpful in defining a truly non-functional incidentaloma as well as unilateral versus bilateral subclinical hypercorticolism.

Hypertension co-existent in patients with bilateral incidentalomas presents an additional diagnostic challenge. The possibility arises of bilateral non-functioning tumours, a non-functioning tumour on one side and a Conn's tumour on the other or bilateral adrenocortical hyperplasia not requiring surgery at all. Selective venous sampling from each adrenal vein for aldosterone and cortisol have been shown[14] to successfully resolve the conundrum and is more reliable than aldosterone postural studies and imaging with thin slice CT or NP-59 scintigraphy.

Key points for clinical practice

- Endoscopic adrenalectomy is the new 'gold' standard for 60% of patients requiring adrenalectomy.

- Transperitoneal and retroperitoneal endoscopic adrenalectomy are comparably effective.

- Patients requiring bilateral adrenalectomy for 'end' stage Cushing's syndrome/disease remain surgically challenging whichever approach is used.

- The algorithm for the management of incidentalomas has been refined.

- Advances in scanning techniques and hormonal assays plus or minus selective venous sampling provide a level of diagnostic accuracy and anatomical localization, etc. which has never before been achieved.

References

1. Geoghegan JG, Emberton M, Bloom SR, Lynn JA. Changing trends in the management of phaeochromocytoma. Br J Surg 1998; 85: 117–120.
2. Nash PA, Leibovitch I, Donohue JP. Adrenalectomy via the dorsal approach: a benchmark for laparoscopic adrenalectomy. J Urol 1995; 154: 1652–1654.
3. Gagner M, Lacroix A, Prinz RA et al Early experience with laparoscopic approach for adrenalectomy. Surgery 1993; 114: 1120–1125.
4. Gagner M, Pomp A, Heniford BT, Pharand D, Lacroix A. Laparoscopic adrenalectomy: lessons learned from 100 consecutive procedures. Ann Surg 1997; 226: 238–246.
5. Thompson GB, Grant CS, van Heerden JA et al. Laparoscopic versus open posterior adrenalectomy: a case-control study of 100 patients. Surgery 1997; 122: 1132–1136.
6. Dudley NE, Harrison BJ. Comparison of open posterior versus transperitoneal laparoscopic adrenalectomy. Br J Surg 1999; 86: 656–660.
7. Staren ED, Prinz RA. Adrenalectomy in the era of laparoscopy. Surgery 1996; 120: 706–711.
8. Bonjer HJ, Lange JF, Kaemier G et al. Comparison of three tecnhiques for adrenalectomy. Br J Surg 1997; 87: 679–682.
9. Duh QY, Siperstein AE, Clark OH et al. Laparoscopic adrenalectomy: comparison of the lateral and posterior approaches. Arch Surg 1996; 131: 870–875.
10. Bencsik ZS, Szabolcs I, Goth M. Incidentally detected adrenal tumours (incidentalomas): histological heterogeneity and differentiated therapeutic approach. J Intern Med 1995; 237: 585–589.
11. Rutherford JC, Gordon RD, Stowasser M et al. Laparoscopic adrenalectomy for adrenal tumours causing hypertension and for 'incidentaloma' of the adrenal on computerized tomography scanning. Clin Exp Pharmacol Physiol 1995; 22: 490–492.
12. Caplan RH, Strutt PJ, Wickus GG. Subclinical hormone secretion by incidentally discovered adrenal masses. Arch Surg 1994; 129: 291–296.
13. Bardet S, Rohmer V, Mucat A et al. ^{131}I-6-Beta-iodomethyl-norcholesterol scintigraphy: an assessment of its role in the investigation of adrenocortical incidentalomas. Clin Endocrinol 1996; 44: 587–596.
14. Young Jr WF, Stanson AW, Grant CS et al. Primary aldosteronism: adrenal venous sampling. Surgery 1996; 120: 913–919.

Brian Birch   Prakash Ratan

Management of benign prostatic hyperplasia

The prostate is present in all mammals but only two – man and dog – develop pathological changes. Why this should be so is unclear. The prostate grows in a linear fashion to 20 years of age, stabilizes and then resumes growth at the age of 50 years onwards[1] making benign prostatic hyperplasia (BPH) the most common neoplastic disease seen in men.[2]

Nearly all men will develop BPH, but the degree of benign prostatic enlargement is variable.[3] Galloway[4] estimates that 14% of 40–49-year-olds and 40% of 70–79-year-olds will have urinary tract symptoms due to BPH. The magnitude of the problem is thus seen to be considerable and is set to increase given that the world population of people aged over 65 years will rise from 390 million now to 800 million by 2025 (World Health Report 1998). Currently, it is estimated in the US alone that more than $4 billion is spent on the medical management of BPH and $2 billion on surgical treatment.[5] In the UK, the management of BPH consumes 0.4% of National Health Service expenditure.[5]

TERMINOLOGY

Historically, urinary symptoms in the older man have been referred to as prostatism or symptomatic BPH. However, urinary symptoms are not specific for BPH, obstruction or even men – occurring as frequently in females. Furthermore, BPH is a histological diagnosis and terms such as prostatism and BPH carry a spurious diagnostic authority. An alternative to these terms proposed by Abrams[6] is lower urinary tract symptoms (LUTS).

Benign prostatic obstruction (BPO) is the condition most urologists want to treat and assumes that attempts have been made to exclude carcinoma. We can then refer to lower urinary tract symptoms suggestive of benign prostatic obstruction in those men who might formerly have been termed as having prostatism.

Mr Brian Birch MA MD FRCS, Consultant Urologist, Southampton University Hospitals Trust, Tremona Road, Southampton SO16 6YD, UK (for correspondence)
Dr Prakash Ratan FRCS, Associate Specialist, Department of Urology, Southampton University Hospitals Trust, Tremona Road, Southampton SO16 6YD, UK

DIAGNOSIS

HISTORY AND SYMPTOM SCORES

There exist many questionnaires designed to evaluate lower urinary tract symptoms in men. However, one must not forget that they are simply tools to measure subjective symptoms and quality of life objectively. The score that usually results from such an exercise lends the findings a spurious mathematical precision. Nevertheless, the finding that as symptom scores increase quality of life decreases[7] lends validity to their use. Furthermore, they allow for comparison between patients and assessments of response to treatment.

The International Prostate Symptom Score (IPSS) is one of the most widely used questionnaires and comprises a seven question set. Each question can produce a score of 0–5, producing a total score lying between 0–35. Symptoms may then be classified as mild (total score 0–7), moderate (8–19) or severe (20–35). There is one further question on the impact of symptoms on the patient's quality of life. Taking a history the urologist should be aware that the main concerns of the patient are:[7,8] (i) lack of sleep; (ii) the symptoms will get worse; (iii) they may have carcinoma; and (iv) the interruption to their daily activities caused by their symptoms.

Thus, while a careful history is obligatory, questionnaires are optional and indeed not used by all urologists.[5] The rationale for this is the claim that symptom indices do not add to management. It is impact of symptoms on quality of life which is more relevant and more predictive of outcome.

Key point 1

- Whilst in general lower urinary tract symptoms in patients over 55 years of age are likely to be due to benign prostatic hyperplasia, in men under 50 years of age alternative diagnoses should be entertained.

EXAMINATION

This is obligatory and includes an abdominal examination, an assessment of peri-anal sensation and a digital rectal examination to identify prostatic abnormalities, including carcinoma. Volume may also be crudely assessed in the knowledge that bigger prostates (greater than 30 ml) show an increased risk of acute urinary retention.[9]

INVESTIGATIONS

Obligatory

It is essential to exclude infection (mid-stream urine analysis), glycosuria secondary to diabetes (dipstick) and haematuria as a possible indication of urinary tract malignancy (MSU or dipstick). In men with marked storage symptoms (frequency, urgency, nocturia) and painful voiding, cytology should be performed and cystoscopy considered.

Recommended

Uroflow: a measurement of the maximum urinary flow rate (Q-max) on two occasions is important. A low Q-max of < 10 ml/s is more likely to be obstructive and treatment failure is more probable (29.4% versus 8.5%) if the maximum flow rate is > 15 ml/s.[5] Interpretations of flow where the voided volume is less than 150 ml is difficult, but persistently low voided volumes themselves are often (72%) indicative of BPO.[10]

Key point 2

- In spite of its limitations, uroflow testing is still the best non-invasive measurement of benign prostatic obstruction.

Post micturition residual volume (PMRV): Measurement of the volume of urine in the bladder after micturition can be assessed non-invasively using ultrasound. Normal men have residual volumes of < 12 ml. Additionally, it has been assumed that an increase in residual urine is evidence of bladder outflow obstruction but it should be regarded as indicating a bladder functional abnormality rather than BPO[5] and grossly elevated residual urine may be associated with neurological disease and an increased risk of upper urinary tract dilatation and renal failure. Men with a large residual urine who opt for non-surgical treatment should be monitored closely as they are at increased risk of developing urinary retention and detrusor failure.

Prostate specific antigen (PSA): Previously, the use of PSA testing in men with LUTS suggestive of BPO was regarded as optional or not recommended. Given the desire of patients and their physicians to exclude carcinoma the routine use of such a test can be justified although there is no clear evidence to link LUTS with an increased risk for prostate cancer.[11]

Optional

Pressure flow studies (PFS): The cystometrogram (CMG) is a non-invasive way of assessing lower urinary tract function. With intravesical and rectal transducers monitoring total bladder (TBP) and intra-abdominal pressure (IAP), respectively, detrusor pressure (DP) can be derived from these two measures (DP = TBP–IAP).

The filling phase of the CMG can yield valuable information concerning bladder capacity, bladder sensation, compliance and the presence of unstable contractions. Pressure flow studies obtained during the voiding phase of the CMG can be correlated with outflow obstruction and represent the only way of distinguishing between low flow secondary to BPO and detrusor failure.

While the necessity for pressure flow studies in the routine management of patients might be debated, they are strongly recommended[12] before offering invasive treatment to men especially those with: (i) a preceding history of neurological disease, e.g. Parkinson's disease or stroke; or (ii) a normal or technically unsatisfactory flow rate. Their use is also justified, in part, by the consideration that in men with LUTS, 25% do not have BPO and 7% with a normal flow are obstructed.

Not recommended

Imaging the upper tracts is not required unless there is a history of stones, haematuria, renal failure/increased creatinine or urinary tract infections.[5]

TREATMENT: PATIENT SELECTION

The paradigm whereby BPH gives rise to benign enlargement of the prostate which in turn results in BPO and LUTS (= symptomatic BPH) is simple and attractive. Before 1992, the job of the primary care physician was to refer patients with prostatism to a competent urologist whose role in patients with sufficient symptoms was to perform a safe transurethral resection of prostate.[13] Studies, unfortunately, have suggested that this attractive idea is too simplistic.

Hald[14] has proposed three concepts requiring consideration in the management of BPH: (i) the presence of prostatic enlargement; (ii) the presence of LUTS; and (iii) urodynamically proven obstruction.

The relationship between these three variables is not straightforward as is well shown using Hald's rings (Fig. 13.1). These show that LUTS and BPO may exist independently of each other and that the presence of one does not necessarily imply the existence of the other; this must not be forgotten in assessing the patient.

Key point 3

- Lower urinary tract symptoms and benign prostatic obstruction may exist independently of each other and that the presence of one does not necessarily imply the existence of the other.

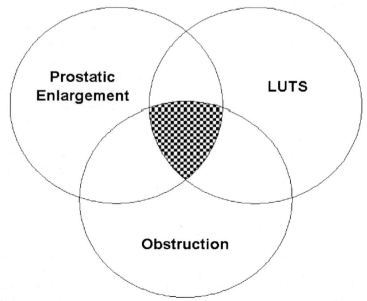

Fig. 13.1 Hald rings. Hatched area = lower urinary tract symptoms (LUTS) due to benign prostatic obstruction (BPO) – formerly known as 'symptomatic' or 'clinical' BPH.

> **Key point 4**
>
> • Treatment is best decided by considering the impact of the disease on quality of life – is this impact mild, moderate or severe. It is this parameter alone that drives the decision making process for patients.

The urologist's aim is to relieve symptoms, reduce BPO and reduce the morbidity secondary to this; worthy goals, but for patients rapid relief of LUTS and increased quality of life (QOL) are more important outcomes.

In general, treatment options fall into three categories: (i) watchful waiting; (ii) medical treatment; and (iii) non-medical treatment (which is invasive to varying degrees).

In the absence of prostate cancer, other lower urinary tract pathology (e.g. interstitial cystitis, bladder cancer) or any absolute indications for surgery (see below) then treatment is best decided by considering the impact of the disease on QOL – is this impact mild, moderate or severe. It is this parameter alone that drives the decision making process for patients.[5]

MILD SYMPTOMS OR BOTHER

In a survey by Gee et al.,[15] the most common treatments chosen by urologists for patients in this category were: (i) watchful waiting; (ii) alpha blockers (21%); and (iii) finasteride (1%). However, the use of phytotherapy in this and other patient groups was not stated and is likely to be significant (see below).

WATCHFUL WAITING

The advantages of watchful waiting are that it has no immediate risks and no side-effects. Barry et al.[16] showed that patients with a diagnosis of BPH had a significant deterioration in symptom scores and flow rates over 2 years. Only 10% improved and acute urinary retention was seen in 5%. These results are similar to those reported by Donovan et al.[17] where patients electing watchful waiting showed no improvement in symptoms. By comparison, the Wasson study[18] showed a failure rate of less than 9% in men with moderate symptoms treated expectantly over a 3 year period. The BAUS guidelines review[12] gives a failure rate for watchful waiting of 38% at 5 years and this may be higher in the type of patients referred to UK urologists. Ultimately, many men are just happy to be re-assured that they are well and do not have prostate cancer.

MODERATE SYMPTOMS OR BOTHER

Gee et al.[15] showed that the most popular treatment of choice amongst urologists for this category of patient was medical treatment – 88% in glands less than 40 ml in size and 69% in glands greater than 40 ml in size. Watchful waiting was used in 3% and finasteride in 1% of cases. Again, no reference was made to phytotherapy.

MEDICAL TREATMENT

Considerable progress has been made in the development of drugs for the treatment of BPO. Although neither patient satisfaction nor the improvement in measurable parameters matches that achieved by transurethral resection of prostate, there is a definite place for medical therapy. The ideal patient for such treatment is one who has mild to moderately bothersome symptoms, no absolute indications for surgery and is willing to undertake a long-term commitment to medication. Three classes of drugs are currently available.

Alpha blockers

It has been variously estimated that 40% of the urethral pressure is due to α-adrenergic tone;[19] understandable given that in the hyperplastic gland the ratio of stroma to epithelium is 5:1 and 29% of the stroma is smooth muscle. This led to the concept of BPO being a two phase model with a static component due to the mechanical effects of the enlarged gland and a dynamic component due to smooth muscle contraction. Alpha blockers would then act to reduce dynamic obstruction.

The α_1-adrenoceptor is the predominant receptor type present in prostate and 98% of these are associated with the stroma. However, molecular cloning studies have identified several sub-types of the α_1-receptor of which the α_{1A} sub-type is the most frequently observed and which increases from 70–85% in BPH.[20] Given that other (α_{1B} and α_{1D}) sub-types are the predominant receptors found on vascular smooth muscle, drugs designed to selectively inhibit the α_{1A} sub-type should have reduced potential for cardiovascular adverse events, e.g. syncope and hypotension. This has proven to be the case with older drugs such as prazosin associated with a less favourable side-effect profile compared with newer drugs, such as tamsulosin and alfuzosin. In general, all α-blockers have similar efficacy and will improve maximum flow rate 20–30% and reduce symptom scores 30–40%.[21] The commonest adverse drug reactions are headache, dizziness, asthenia, and drowsiness with tamsulosin and alfuzosin causing the least problems.[22]

However, the long-term efficacy of α-blockers remains to be established and they do not halt the progression of BPO nor the occurrence of its complications. Also, they do not relieve obstruction on urodynamic studies despite this being a rationale for their use. That α-blockers are effective suggests that they may have other sites of action (e.g. the spinal cord) or act via α_1-adrenergic independent pathways (e.g. to increase apoptosis in the prostate).[23]

Key point 5

- The long-term efficacy of α-blockers remains to be established and they do not halt the progression of benign prostatic obstruction nor the occurrence of its complications.

5-α-reductase inhibitors

Only one drug, finasteride, is currently available. This specifically and competitively inhibits the type 2 isoenzyme of 5-α-reductase and prevents the conversion of testosterone to the more potent androgen dihydrotestosterone. Its use results in a decrease in prostate volume most marked in the epithelial compartment and approximating 15–20%[24] thereby reducing the static component of BPO.

Whilst attractive in theory, finasteride has proven less useful in clinical practice. Lepor et al.[25] have shown that finasteride is inferior to alpha blockade with terazosin and was only superior to placebo in glands greater than 50 ml in volume. Given this, a slow onset of action (at least 3 months) and reported adverse drug reactions (ejaculatory failure 2.1%, reduced libido 1%, gynaecomastia 0.4%) it is not surprising that finasteride is used less frequently than alpha blockers in the treatment of BPO.

More recent data have suggested that long-term treatment with finasteride will reduce the need for transurethral resection of prostate (TURP) and the rate of acute urinary retention by up to 50%. However, the cost of prevention in this fashion exceeds the cost of TURP done at the time of retention and ignores the real sexual side-effects of the drug.[21] Where finasteride has proven useful is in the management of bleeding secondary to BPH. It should also be noted that the use of finasteride will reduce PSA levels, but these can be corrected by the simple expedient of doubling them. In this way surveillance for prostate cancer can be continued if necessary. As finasteride is excreted in the semen it should not be used in heterosexual men with fertile partners.

Phytotherapy

The use of plant extracts to treat LUTS suggestive of BPO is very frequent both in the US ($1.5 billion per year) and continental Europe where it comprises 90% of all drugs prescribed for treatment.[26,27] In such preparations, the standardization of the active ingredients where known is difficult and their mode of action is unclear. A lack of randomized controlled trials further clouds the issue. Of the available preparations *Saw palmetto* (mostly as permixon) is the most frequently used.[27]

Studies generally show little if any changes in objective parameters of BPO but symptoms are improved. Only *Saw palmetto* and β-sitosterols seem to be more effective than placebo with the former having an effect equivalent to finasteride.[28]

SEVERE SYMPTOMS OR BOTHER

Reviews[15] show that alpha blockers still remain the most popular treatment in this category of patient, being used in 45–58% of cases. Transurethral resection of prostate is the next most frequent choice (31–38%). Some urologists use alternative surgical techniques which will also be briefly discussed here. Generally, where invasive techniques are being considered in treatment, the use of pressure flow studies before treatment is recommended. The rationale for this is that treatment outcome is significantly better in men with unequivocal obstruction and normal detrusor function.[29,30]

TRANSURETHRAL RESECTION OF PROSTATE (TURP)

TURP remains the gold standard for the treatment of LUTS suggestive of BPO.[31] However, the wider use of medical treatment has seen falls of up to 60%

in its use (Nickel C., personal communication). The morbidity data used to compare TURP to other less invasive treatments are generally based on data from the late 1980s. More recent studies[32] have shown that TURP in the 1990s has improved considerably and is a safe, well-tolerated and effective treatment. Transfusion is seen in only 0.2% of patients with intra-operative complications in just 2.5% and no mortality. Postoperative complications are seen in 8.5% (mostly urinary tract infection). Both hospital stays and catheter times average less than 1.5 days and the need for repeat TURP was 2.5% with incontinence rates < 1%.

Complications specific to TURP which patients should be counselled about pre-operatively include retrograde ejaculation (70–90%) and impotence (< 5%).

Generally, symptoms improve in approximately 90% of patients and peak flows improve by 125%.[31] Whilst symptoms remain a relative indication for TURP, absolute indications for surgery include acute urinary retention with at least one failed trial without catheter, recurrent gross haematuria, bladder stones and renal insufficiency secondary to BPO.

TRANSURETHRAL INCISION OF THE PROSTATE (TUIP)

Whereas TURP aims to remove adenomatous obstructing prostatic tissue, in TUIP one (or two) relaxing incisions are made in the bladder neck/prostate out to the capsule. This has the advantage of being quicker than TURP and has a lower morbidity. Retrograde ejaculation is seen less frequently (up to 50%). Previously TUIP has been recommended as an alternative to TURP in smaller (less than 40 g) glands. However, more recent studies[33] suggest that TURP is the superior treatment.

LASER TRANSURETHRAL RESECTION OF PROSTATE

Four types of laser can be used to treat the prostate: neodymium-YAG, holmium-YAG, KTP-YAG and diode. The energy can be delivered through a bare fibre (contact), right angle fibre or interstitial fibre. Coagulation is seen at temperatures of 65°C and vaporization when temperature changes exceed 100°C. In general, better results are achieved with contact laser techniques – which result in vaporization and tissue resection – compared to coagulation techniques using right-angled fibres. Enthusiasts point to reduced blood loss and short catheter times compared with TURP, but with modern techniques such differences are small and for an experienced resectionist a laser TURP, especially in the larger gland, can be a somewhat tedious experience. Improvements in symptom scores are not dissimilar to TURP but relief of obstruction is less impressive.[34]

Interstitial laser coagulation involves the placement under direct vision of a fibre in the prostatic stroma via a puncture in the prostatic urethra. It induces coagulation necrosis and its main disadvantage is prolonged postoperative catheterization in the order of 7–21 days.[35]

Transurethral needle ablation (TUNA)

TUNA is a technique whereby low radiofrequency waves are used to heat the prostate via needles introduced into the prostatic stroma under direct vision.

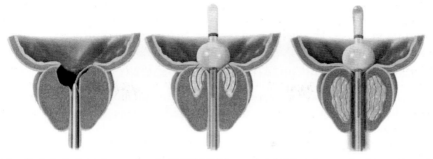

Fig. 13.2 Left: initial resection in TURP. Middle and right: two types of microwave hyperthermia – that in the middle being directed at the bladder neck and that to the left against the lateral lobes.

Coagulative necrosis results. Postoperative retention is seen in 13–42% of patients and irritative lower urinary tract symptoms in 40% lasting up to 1 week. Flow rates are improved but less than with TURP and 73% are still obstructed at 2 years.[36]

TRANSURETHRAL MICROWAVE THERMOTHERAPY (TUMT)

This involves the use of systems designed to deliver microwaves to the prostate (Fig. 13.2). The energy generated by the microwaves is absorbed and converted to thermal energy resulting in hyperthermia (42–44°C), thermotherapy (> 45°C) or thermal ablation (> 70°C). As might be expected, the results of early delivery systems using low temperatures transrectally are inferior to those using the transurethral route with higher radiant energy and water conductive cooling to preserve the urethral epithelium. The most effective of the latter type of devices include the high energy Prostatron

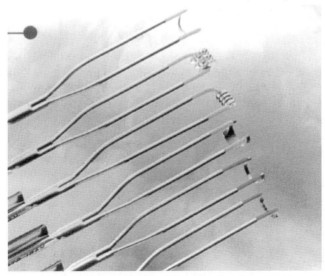

Fig. 13.3 Range of vaporization electrodes. The spiked and grooved configurations can be seen second and third from the top, respectively.

machine using Prostasoft software version 2.5 and the Targis device from Urologix. Flow rates increase in the order of 38% are seen with a 50% reduction in symptom scores. The majority of patients (79%) remain obstructed.[34]

TRANSURETHRAL VAPORIZATION OF THE PROSTATE (TUVP)

TUVP allows simultaneous vaporization and coagulation using a range of electrodes (Fig. 13.3). Generally, these are configured as grooved or spiked rollers that allow both an increased number of edges where high current densities result in vaporization of tissue and wide contact areas elsewhere which give rise to coagulation. Similar instrumentation is used to TURP (the only change being a substitution of the electrode for the transurethral resection loop) with the cutting current increased by 25–75%.[37]

Preliminary results are encouraging with reductions in symptom scores and rates of retrograde ejaculation similar to TURP but with more postoperative irritation and less relief of obstruction.[34] Erectile dysfunction may be slightly higher with TUVP (17% compared with 11% for TURP),[38] but incontinence is not a problem to date.

OPEN PROSTATECTOMY

Performed via the retropubic or transvesical routes, open prostatectomy improves lower urinary tract symptoms in 98% of patients with increases in maximum flow rates of around 175%. Bladder neck stenosis, impotence, urethral stricture and retrograde ejaculation are all more common than with TURP.[31] Postoperative complications are also more common with longer postoperative hospitalization. It is generally reserved for very large glands in excess of 150–200 g and patients with hip problems preventing adequate positioning for TURP.

MISCELLANEOUS TREATMENTS

Stents
Permanent stents (which become epithelialized) and temporary stents have been used as flexible prostheses placed into the prostatic urethra to hold it open. Although theoretically attractive as an alternative to long-term catheterization in the elderly and infirm, the risks of displacement, infection, incontinence, calcification and encrustation detracts from the merit of their use. Furthermore, obstruction is not relieved[34] and, as such, stenting has failed to gain wide-spread acceptance.

Balloon dilatation
This uses a special balloon catheter inserted transurethrally to dilate the prostatic urethra. Obstruction is not relieved and there is a feeling that the benefits are placebo-related and short-lived. It has fallen from favour.

Emerging technologies
Further techniques under evaluation in the treatment of LUTS suggestive of BPO include: (i) high intensity focused ultrasound mounted on a transurethral

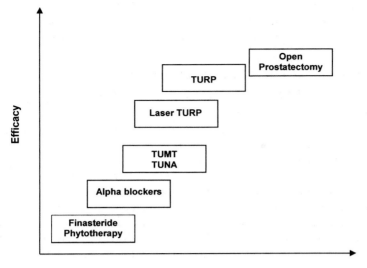

Fig. 13.4 Comparison of efficacies and complications of BPH treatments. TUMT, transurethral microwave thermotherapy; TUNA, transurethral needle ablation of the prostate; TURP, transurethral resection of the prostate.

catheter delivery system (preliminary results show outcomes similar to TUMP or TUNA); (ii) transurethral injection of alcohol; and (iii) transurethral enzymatic ablation using hyaluronidase and collagenase.

CONCLUSIONS

Despite the varying success of the aforementioned treatments for LUTS suggestive of BPO, their exact mode of action is unclear. What is clear is that obstruction does not have to be relieved for symptoms to be improved, suggesting a neurological target for such techniques. We rather suspect that the relatively greater success of more invasive treatments is not due solely to the fact that they reduce the static component of obstruction by reducing the physical size of the prostate, but also because they too have a neurological target possibly at the level of the micturition reflex.

It is clear that the treatment offered to a patient should match his perceptions of the impact of the disease on his quality of life, i.e. the patient should be treated not his flow rate.

Trends in the use of various techniques give some insight as to how treatment is developing or evolving in the management of BPO. Thus, the number of urologists using non-contact laser prostatectomy has fallen from 42% to 26% in the US and the number using contact laser techniques has similarly fallen from 45% to 26%. TURP remains popular at 95% and both TUMT and TUNA are only used by a small number of practitioners (3% each). However, the rate of TUVP has increased from 54% to 62%.[15]

TURP remains the gold standard of treatment for the time being and the durability and success from surgery is clear – 90% of patients do not require a

Key points for clinical practice

- Whilst in general lower urinary tract symptoms in patients over 55 years of age are likely to be due to benign prostatic hyperplasia, in men under 50 years of age alternative diagnoses should be entertained.

- In spite of its limitations, uroflow testing is still the best non-invasive measurement of benign prostatic obstruction.

- Lower urinary tract symptoms and benign prostatic obstruction may exist independently of each other and that the presence of one does not necessarily imply the existence of the other.

- Treatment is best decided by considering the impact of the disease on quality of life – is this impact mild, moderate or severe. It is this parameter alone that drives the decision making process for patients.

- The long-term efficacy of α-blockers remains to be established and they do not halt the progression of benign prostatic obstruction nor the occurrence of its complications.

- Transurethral resection of prostate remains the gold standard of treatment for the time being and the durability and success from surgery is clear – 90% of patients do not require a second operation and 80–90% have symptomatic relief..

second operation and 80–90% have symptomatic relief. No other treatment, with the exception of open prostatectomy has been shown to be as effective (see Fig. 13.4).[39] Given that modern day TURP is not as invasive a treatment as it used to be, there are many (including the authors) who feel that its use should be more wide-spread.

References

1. Berry SJ, Coffey DS, Walsh PC, Ewing LL. The development of benign prostatic hyperplasia with age. J Urol 1984; 132: 474–479.
2. Walsh PC. Benign prostatic hyperplasia: etiological considerations. Prog Clin Biol Res 1984; 145: 1–25.
3. Lepor H. The pathophysiology of lower urinary tract symptoms in the ageing male population. Br J Urol 1998; 81 (Suppl 1): 29–33.
4. Garraway WM, Collins GN, Lee RJ. High prevalence of benign prostatic hypertrophy in the community. Lancet 1991; 338: 469–471.
5. Jepsen JV, Bruskewitz RC. Office evaluation of men with lower urinary tract symptoms. Urol Clin North Am 1998; 25: 545–554.
6. Abrams P. New words for old: lower urinary tract symptoms for 'prostatism'. BMJ 1994; 308: 929–930.
7. Trueman P, Hood SC, Nayak USL, Mrazek MF. Prevalence of lower urinary tract symptoms and self reported diagnosed benign prostatic hyperplasia , and their effect on quality of life in a community-based survey of men in the UK. BJU Int 1999; 83: 410–415.
8. Da Silva FC, Marquis P, Deschaseaux P et al. Relative importance of sexuality and quality of life in patients with prostatic symptoms. Results of an international study. Eur Urol 1997; 31: 272–280.

9. Williams G. Other assessments: prostate size and prostate specific antigen. BJU Int 2000; 85 (Suppl 1): 31–35.

10. Reynard JM, Yang Q, Donovan JL et al. The ICS-'BPH' study: uroflowmetry, lower urinary tract symptoms and bladder outlet obstruction. Br J Urol 1998; 82: 619–623.

11. Young JM, Muscatello DJ, Ward JE. Are men with lower urinary tract symptoms at increased risk of prostate cancer? A systematic review and critique of the available evidence. BJU Int 2000; 85: 1037–1048.

12. Bradshaw C, Donovan JL, George NJR et al. Guidelines on the Management of Men with Lower Urinary Tract Symptoms suggesting Bladder Outflow Obstruction. London: The Royal College of Surgeons of England and The British Association of Urological Surgeons. January 1997.

13. Lieber MM. Pharmacologic therapy for prostatism. Mayo Clin Proc 1998; 73: 590–596.

14. Hald T. Urodynamics in benign prostatic hyperplasia: a survey. Prostate Suppl 1989; 2: 69–77.

15. Gee WF, Holtgrewe HL, Blute ML et al. 1997 American Urological Association Gallup Survey: changes in the diagnosis and management of prostate cancer and benign prostatic hyperplasia, and other practice trends from 1994 to 1997. J Urol 1998; 160: 1804–1807.

16. Barry MJ, Fowler Jr FJ, Bin L et al. The natural history of patients with benign prostatic hyperplasia as diagnosed by North American urologists. J Urol 1997; 157: 10–15.

17. Donovan JL, Brookes ST, de la Rosette JJ et al. The responsiveness of the ICSmale questionnaire to outcome: evidence from the ICS-'BPH' study. BJU Int 1999; 83: 243–248.

18. Wasson JH, Reda DJ, Bruskewitz RC et al. A comparison of transurethral surgery with watchful waiting for moderate symptoms of benign prostatic hyperplasia. N Engl J Med 1995; 332: 75–79.

19. Beduschi MC, Beduschi R, Oesterling JE. Alpha-blockade therapy for benign prostatic hyperplasia: from a non-selective to a more selective alpha 1A-adrenergic antagonist. Urology 1998; 51: 861–872.

20. Kawabe K. Current status of research on prostate-selective alpha 1-antagonists. Br J Urol 1998; 81 (Suppl 1): 48–50.

21. Chapple CR. Medical therapy and quality of life. Eur Urol 1998; 34 (Suppl 2): 10–17.

22. Chapple CR. Pharmacotherapy for benign prostatic hyperplasia – the potential for alpha 1-adrenoceptor subtype-specific blockade. Br J Urol 1998; 81 (Suppl 1): 34–47.

23. Fitzpatrick JM. Facts and future lines of research in lower urinary tract symptoms in men and women: an overview of the role of alpha 1-adrenoreceptor antagonists. BJU Int 2000; 85 (Suppl 2): 1–5.

24. Wilde MI, Goa KL. Finasteride. An update of its use in the management of symptomatic benign prostatic hyperplasia. Drugs 1999; 57: 557–581.

25. Lepor H, Williford WO, Barry MJ et al. The impact of medical therapy on bother due to symptoms, quality of life and global outcome, and factors predicting response. J Urol 1998; 160: 1358–1367.

26. Wilt TJ, Ishami A, Stark G et al. *Saw palmetto* extracts for treatment of benign prostatic hyperplasia. JAMA 1998; 280: 1604–1609.

27. Gerber GS. *Saw palmetto* for the treatment of men with lower urinary tract symptoms. J Urol 2000; 163: 1408–1412.

28. Lowe FC, Fegelman E. Phytotherapy in the treatment of benign prostatic hyperplasia: an update. Urology 1999; 53: 671–678.

29. Javlé P, Jenkins SA, Machin DG, Parsons KF. Grading of benign prostatic obstruction can predict the outcome of transurethral prostatectomy. J Urol 1998; 160: 1713–1717.

30. Roehrborn CG, Burkhard FC, Bruskewitz RC et al. The effects of transurethral needle ablation and resection of the prostate on pressure flow urodynamic parameters: analysis of the United States randomised study. J Urol 1999; 162: 92–97.

31. Jepsen JV, Bruskewitz RC. Recent developments in the surgical management of benign prostatic hyperplasia. Urology 1998; 51 (Suppl 4A): 23–31.

32. Borboroglu PG, Kane CJ, Ward JF et al. Immediate and postoperative complications of transurethral prostatectomy in the 1990s. J Urol 1999; 162: 1307–1310.

33. Jahnson S, Dalén M, Gustavsson G, Pedersen J. Transurethral incision versus resection of the prostate for small to medium benign prostatic hyperplasia. Br J Urol 1998; 81: 276–281.

34. Ruud Bosch JLH. Urodynamic effect of various treatment modalities for benign prostatic hyperplasia . J Urol 1997; 158: 2034–2044.
35. Perlmutter AP, Muschter R. Interstitial laser prostatectomy. Mayo Clin Proc 1998; 73: 903–907.
36. Chapple CR, Issa MM, Woo H. Transurethral needle ablation (TUNA). A clinical review of radiofrequency thermal therapy in the management of benign prostatic hyperplasia. Eur Urol 1999; 35: 119–128.
37. Weiner DM, Kaplan SA. Electrosurgery: VaporTrode. Eur Urol 1999; 35: 166–172.
38. Hammadeh MY, Madaan S, Singh M, Philp T. Two year follow-up of a prospective randomised trial electrovaporization versus resection of the prostate. Eur Urol 1998; 34: 188–192.
39. Fitzpatrick JM. A critical evaluation of technological innovations in the treatment of symptomatic benign prostatic hyperplasia. Br J Urol 1998; 81 (Suppl 1): 56–63.

Jagdeep Chana   Paul Tulley

CHAPTER 14

Surgical aspects of the management of skin tumours

This review will concentrate on the surgical aspects of management of the three commonest cutaneous carcinomas which include basal cell carcinoma, squamous cell carcinoma and malignant melanoma. The basic principles regarding reconstruction following excision of these tumours are also discussed.

BASAL CELL CARCINOMA

A number of histological varieties of basal cell carcinoma (BCC) exist with 26 varieties being identified in one series.[1] However, most tumours fall into one of the following histological types: (i) nodular-ulcerative; (ii) morphoeic; (iii) pigmented; (iv) superficial; (v) field-fire; (vi) cystic; or (vii) infiltrative. The treatment of BCC falls within three broad categories which include surgical, destructive and radiotherapy.

SURGICAL EXCISION

Surgical excision is the most common form of treatment with an overall cure rate of 91%.[2] The likelihood of cure decreases with the size of lesion. Epstein reported that visual assessment of the margins of BCC was within 1 mm of the actual border in 94% of cases and this observation led him to believe that a 2 mm excision margin gave a 94% cure rate.[3] Wolf and Zitelli have found that for tumours with a diameter of < 2 cm, a minimum margin of 4 mm was necessary for total excision in 94% of cases.[4] Therefore, most authors currently recommend margins of 5 mm when excising BCCs of small nodular subtype. However, cure rates sharply decline when dealing with larger tumours, or those with infiltrative or morphoeic morphology. In Sexton et al.'s analysis of

Mr Jagdeep Chana BSc MD FRCS, Specialist Registrar in Plastic Surgery, Mount Vernon Hospital, Northwood, Middlesex HA6 2RN, UK (for correspondence)
Mr Paul Tulley BSc FRCS, RAFT Research Fellow, RAFT Institute of Plastic Surgery, Northwood, Middlesex HA6 2RN, UK

1039 BCCs, nodular and superficial BCCs were completely excised in 93.6% and 96.4% of cases, whereas infiltrative and morphoeic types had an incomplete excision rate of 26.5% and 33.3%, respectively.[5]

MOHS' MICROGRAPHIC SURGERY

Mohs' micrographic surgery involves excision of all the visible tumour in horizontal slices while mapping the exact size and shape of the lesion. Horizontal frozen sections are taken from the undersurface of the excised lesion and are examined microscopically. Incompletely excised areas of tumour are mapped and marked for further excision. This process is repeated until the entire tumour is removed. The advantages of this technique for excision of skin tumours are high cure rates, decreased morbidity, and tissue conservation. The only disadvantage is the need for two separate procedures when reconstruction is required. In many cases, conventional frozen section can be just as effective in detecting residual tumour foci. The indications for Mhos' micrographic surgery are outlined by Cottel.[6]

DESTRUCTIVE TREATMENTS

Destructive treatments for BCC include electrodessication and curettage (EDC), cryosurgery and CO_2 laser.

EDC is a common method for treatment of BCC with reported cure rates of as high as 96–100%.[7] However, when analysed by tumour size it is evident that this form of treatment is effective for only very small tumours. Lesions less than 2 mm are completely removed 100% of the time, lesions of 2–5 mm are removed in 85% of cases and tumours >3 cm recur in 50% of cases.[2] This technique is, therefore, recommended only for very small and superficial tumours.[2].

Similarly, cryosurgery is an acceptable form of treatment for small tumours. The study by Zacarian based on his experience of 4228 tumours achieved a cure rate of 97.4% but only 10% of his tumours were >2 cm.[8] Complications of treatment with cryosurgery include marked oedema, a long period of morbidity, and permanent hypopigmentation at the site of treatment. Cryosurgery is, therefore, best reserved for small lesions.

The CO_2 laser produces superficial vaporisation of tissue in a very controlled manner limiting adjacent thermal damage. It is useful in treating superficial BCCs that are confined to the epidermis and papillary dermis only.[9] Appropriate treatment usually requires three passes on clinically visible tumour with treatment of at least 4 mm of surrounding healthy skin.[10] Laser treatment of tumours extending deeper than the epidermis or superficial papillary dermis is inappropriate because of scarring and the inability to assess the margins of the residual tumour. Laser is particularly useful in treating patients with multiple tumours and especially patients with the hereditary Gorlins' syndrome who present with numerous BCC tumours. As with all non-surgical methods, the disadvantage of laser treatment is the inability to examine pathological margins.

Radiotherapy can be used to treat BCC and an overall cure rate of 92% has been reported in the treatment of skin malignancies.[2] The disadvantages of radiotherapy are the prolonged duration of treatment and, although there are few cosmetic defects initially, the results deteriorate over time with fibrosis, telangectasia, ectropion and ulceration. There is even a risk of radiation osteitis and chondritis on treatment of certain areas. Radiation should, therefore, be reserved for elderly patients who are not suitable candidates for surgery.

In the incompletely excised BCC, the options are re-excision or observation. A number of authors estimate that approximately one-third of all incompletely excised BCCs will recur.[11–14] In one study it was found that when the tumour is within one high-power field of the surgical margin, 12% of the lesions recurred whereas a 33% recurrence rate exists when tumour actually involves the surgical margin.[15] Of the 30% of patients with incompletely excised BCC whose lesions recur, 85% have a recurrence within 3 years of surgery.[16] Other authors report a lower recurrence rate with only 66% of lesions returning in the first 3 years.[17] Although these recurrence rates have prompted some surgeons to observe patients with incompletely excised BCC, Koplin and Zarem recommend immediate re-excision of all lesions with positive margins.[18]

SQUAMOUS CELL CARCINOMA

The treatment of cutaneous squamous cell carcinoma (SCC) is similar to BCC and may involve surgical excision, destructive therapy or radiotherapy. The choice of treatment is influenced by tumour size, location, extent of invasion of neighbouring structures, as well as patient age, general health and cosmetic requirements. SCC is more aggressive than BCC and, therefore, wider excision margins are required for local control.

In 95% of cases of well differentiated SCC <2 cm in diameter, a 4 mm margin is adequate .[19] Larger tumours require a 1 cm margin.[20] Recurrence rates of SCC after surgical excision are 5–6%.[21] As the tumour size increases, the likelihood of cure diminishes because the margins needed to guarantee complete excision become excessively wide. If the treatment of a 3 cm tumour is to have 75% chance of cure, the surgical margin must be 1.7 cm, but to achieve a 95% chance of cure a 3.5 cm margin is necessary.[22]

Mohs' micrographic technique has also been used for SCC. Mohs reported a 94% cure in primary cutaneous SCC.[23]. Although the advantages of this technique are tissue preservation and lower recurrence rates, the disadvantages are considerable patient inconvenience and expense. Destructive techniques such as cryosurgery and electrodessication and curettage do not produce a surgical specimen for histological and margin analysis. Additionally, healing is by secondary intention, which results in poorer scars than if the wound is closed primarily. Destructive techniques are, therefore, best reserved for small superficial lesions in non-critical areas as the local failure rate is high. Radiotherapy has been shown to cure SCC in 90% of cases.[24] However, the side-effects can be unpleasant and the treatment protracted; therefore, this modality is best reserved for the debilitated patient who is a poor surgical candidate or for the patient who refuses surgery.[21] Radiotherapy is, however, an effective adjuvant treatment in high stage large tumours or recurrent tumours. Topical 5-fluorouracil (5-FU) is an excellent method of treating premalignant lesions associated with SCC, such as actinic keratoses, but it is not recommended for the primary treatment of squamous carcinoma.

Surgical aspects of the management of skin tumours

SCC has a metastatic potential with the risk of metastases for lesions on the trunk or extremities ranging from 2–5%. Lesions of the face or the dorsum of the hand have a higher metastatic rate, between 10–20%. The risk of regional lymphatic spread from cutaneous SCC is less than that of mucosal SCC.[21] Patients with regional recurrence require a lymphadenectomy.[19] However, the role of prophylactic lymph node dissection is unclear.[25]

MELANOMA

Surgery has remained the treatment modality of choice for primary cutaneous melanoma throughout this century. Until 1977 extremely wide margins were used for melanoma excision. However, in 1977, Breslow and Macht suggested that conservative excision margins would be adequate in melanomas less than 0.76 mm in depth,[26] but there was no evidence at that time this had no effect on recurrence rate or survival through prospective randomised trials.

In 1979, the World Health Organization (WHO) Melanoma Programme commenced a large prospective multicentre trial comparing excision margins of 1 cm and 3 cm in tumours less than 2 mm thick. A total of 612 patients were evaluable in this trial and matched for age, sex, tumour thickness and site as part of the randomisation process. At publication, the median follow-up was 100 months and there was no significant difference in overall survival between the two groups.[27] This study, therefore, concluded that an excision margin of 1 cm was safe for tumours less than 2 mm thick. Subsequent analysis revealed a slight difference in recurrence rate for tumours 1–2 mm thick treated by the two widths of excision. Five local recurrences were observed in the group with the narrow margin (tumours 1–2 mm thick) compared to one local recurrence in the group having the wider margin. The results were, therefore, inconclusive for tumours between 1–2 mm in thickness. However, the overall recurrence rate whichever margin was applied remained very low at 3%.[28] The results of this trial indicate that most melanomas below 2 mm in depth can be treated as an out-patient procedure with a l cm excision margin under local anaesthetic.

A subsequent multi-institutional study randomised 486 patients with intermediate thickness lesions between 1–4 mm on the trunk and extremities to excisions with margins of either 2 cm or 4 cm.[29] No significant difference was found in the rate of local recurrence or in-transit metastases (metastases between the excision and the regional nodal basin). Recurrence rates in both groups did not correlate with surgical margins even among stratified thickness groups. The need for skin grafting was reduced from 47% with 4 cm margins to 11% with 2 cm margins. These data led to a reduction in margins of excision for intermediate-thickness (1–4 mm) lesions to 2 cm.

Future data will no doubt add greater precision to the appropriateness of specific margins of excision. In cosmetically and functionally vital regions, such as the eyes, ears, or mouth and on the digits, the revision and reduction of uniformly wide excision margins have allowed more cosmetically and functionally optimal surgery.

At the present time, reasonable guidelines for appropriate margins of excision for cutaneous malignant melanoma would be:[30]

1. Malignant melanoma in situ: excisions with 0.5 cm margins to ensure complete ablation.

2,   Lesions classified as <1 mm in thickness: conservative excisions with margins no greater than 1 cm, thereby allowing a primary closure in virtually all instances.

3,   Intermediate-thickness lesions (1–4 mm): 2 cm margins are appropriate.

4.   Thick lesions (> 4 mm): margins wider than 2 cm may be required to optimise local control.

Currently, the question of conservative excision for tumours greater than 2 mm in depth is being addressed by a combined study organised by The Melanoma Study Group (MSG) and the British Association of Plastic Surgeons (BAPS) to investigate the effect of 1 cm versus 3 cm excision. The conservative approach to excision margins has also affected the management of melanoma in situ with evidence suggesting that 0.5 cm is adequate if reliable histology has proven that the basement membrane was not breached.[31]

MANAGEMENT OF REGIONAL LYMPH NODE METASTASES

Surgical excision remains the treatment of choice for clinically involved regional lymph nodes. The techniques of block dissection remain the same as for other malignancies. Morbidity is greater after inguinal than after axillary dissection. Trimming back skin flaps before closure and transposing the sartorius muscle to cover the femoral vessels can reduce wound complications. In a report of 168 patients undergoing inguinal dissections at the MD Anderson Cancer Center, wound problems occurred in 20% of cases and were related to age (over 50 years) and smoking.[32] Besides anecdotal reports, there is no convincing evidence that survival is altered after radical ilio-obturator lymph node dissection (RID) relative to superficial femoral dissection (SFD). However, in a retrospective study of 133 patients at the Royal Marsden Hospital, groin recurrence was significantly more frequent after SFD (57.1%) than after RID (23.3 %).[33]

In contrast to the role of therapeutic dissection, the need for elective lymph node dissection (ELND) remains embroiled in controversy. It is postulated that elective dissection of nodes at the time of treatment of the primary tumour will remove micrometastatic deposits which subsequently give rise to clinically overt disease. Although reports from a number of retrospective non-randomised trials have shown a survival advantage following ELND,[34,35] these results have not been demonstrated by two large multicentre prospective trials, both of which have shown no advantage in terms of disease free interval or overall survival.[36,37] Furthermore, the complication rate of this procedure produces considerable morbidity and occasional mortality.

Part of the reason for the failure of ELND to show significant benefit relates to the fact that only 25% of patients having had elective dissection show histological evidence of occult micrometastasis. It is argued by the protagonists of ELND that the possible benefit in the subgroup with proven micrometastasis is diluted by the remaining 75%, who have, in effect, had an unnecessary procedure. To clarify this issue, Cochran and Morton have proposed the method of intra-operative lymphatic mapping and sentinel node biopsy.[38,39]. The method involves identifying the sentinel lymph node, which is the first in the regional chain to drain the area of skin affected by melanoma.

This is performed pre-operatively by lymphoscintigraphy and peri-operatively following intradermal injection of patent-blue dye, which is taken up by the sentinel node. This node is then excised and sent for frozen-section examination whilst the patient is still under anaesthetic. If occult micrometastases are identified, formal block dissection is performed (selective lymph node dissection, SLND). If histology reveals no evidence of tumour, then no dissection is performed and the patient followed up routinely. Early results of this technique have revealed an improvement in survival compared to historical controls.[40] This has prompted a prospective multicentre trial between centres in the US and Australia to investigate the effect of SLND on survival of patients with primary tumours over 1.5 mm in thickness. The results of this trial will hopefully settle some of the arguments raging over the use of adjuvant lymph node dissection.

RECONSTRUCTION FOLLOWING TUMOUR EXCISION

The majority of defects following the excision of small tumours can be closed directly. However, larger defects may require the use of skin grafts or flaps. A skin graft is tissue, usually skin, that is taken from one part of the body and transferred to a secondary site where it must establish a blood supply by the in-growth of new vessels. A flap, however, does not need to establish a blood supply from the recipient bed since it remains attached to the body by a pedicle or it is microvascularly transferred with its supplying blood vessels. A flap can, therefore, be used to cover areas where a graft will not take.

Skin grafts can be used to cover defects following the excision of most skin tumours. A skin graft will not take on exposed cortical bone without periosteum, cartilage without perichondrium, tendon without paratenon, or irradiated tissue. In these situations a flap is required to provide cover. Split thickness grafts do not look like normal skin, as they do not contain the full thickness of the skin or the supporting tissues. They are normally used for situations where urgent cover is required for an otherwise healthy skin defect, or where the appearance is not important. The quality and match of a skin graft depends not only on whether it is partial thickness or full-thickness, but also on whether the graft has a good colour and texture match to the recipient area. For example, a full thickness graft from the post auricular area is an excellent match for the cheek and the lower eyelid when compared to grafts taken from other parts of the body. The choice of the skin graft and the donor site, therefore, depends on aesthetic and functional considerations as well as the size of the area to be covered,

Flaps are used in situations where: (i) grafts will not take; (ii) there is a risk of scar contracture, e.g. across a joint; (iii) the aesthetic result is important; (iv) bulk or structural support is needed; or (iii) transfer of vascularised tissue is specialised, e.g. bone or innervated muscle.

COMMON TYPES OF SKIN FLAPS USED FOR SKIN TUMOUR EXCISION

Flap classifications vary according to the organising principle, whether vascular supply, method of transfer or tissue composition. Flaps may be random or axial pattern according to their blood supply or local or distant. Axial flaps may be pedicled, island or free (microvascular transfer) because of their incorporated blood vessels. Axial flaps can also be cutaneous, fascial, fasciocutaneous, muscle, myocutaneous or osteomyocutaneous. This allows the surgeon to tailor a flap to suit any reconstructive situation.

Local flaps

Common types of local flaps in use are advancement, rotation, transposition, bilobed or rhomboid.

A rotation flap is a semicircular flap of skin and subcutaneous tissue that rotates about a pivot point into the defect to be closed. Its donor site can be closed by a skin graft or by direct closure. To facilitate rotation of the flap along its arc, the base can be back-cut at its base or a triangle of skin (Burrow's triangle) can be removed external to the pivot point (Fig. 14.1).

Advancement flaps are moved directly forward into a defect simply by stretching the skin, without any rotation or lateral movement. Variations are single or double pedicled advancement or V-Y advancement (Fig. 14.2).

A transposition flap is usually a rectangular piece of skin and subcutaneous tissue that is rotated about a pivot point into an immediately adjacent defect. The effective length of the flap becomes shorter the farther it is rotated, the flap must be designed longer than the defect to be covered (Fig. 14.3). The donor site can be closed by skin graft or direct suture. A bilobed flap is a transposition flap where a secondary smaller flap is raised to fill the primary defect (Fig. 14.4). The rhomboid flap is another transposition flap suitable for the closure of rhomboid defects with angles of 60 degrees (Fig. 14.5).

Many of the principles surrounding the use of local flaps can be used together with tissue expansion where new skin is generated by the use of subcutaneously implanted expanders that are then inflated over time to provide skin to cover large defects. This technique has been covered in detail in a previous issue of *Recent Advances in Surgery*.[41]

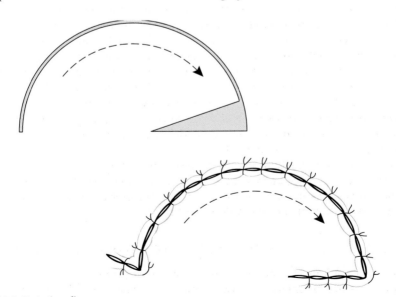

Fig. 14.1 Rotation flap.

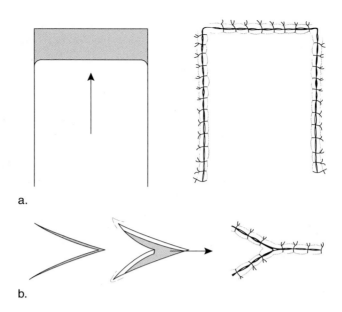

Fig. 14.2 (a) Advancement flap; (b) V-Y advancement flap.

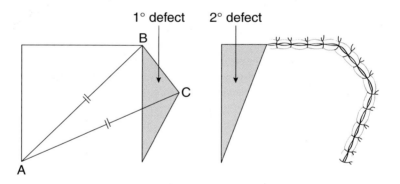

Fig. 14.3 Transposition flap.

Island flaps

These flaps are an axial pattern flap where the skin paddle is entirely detached from the surrounding skin except for a vascular pedicle. This allows the flap much greater mobility as it is not hindered by a skin pedicle. Subcutaneous island flaps consisting only of skin and subcutaneous tissue are useful for head and neck reconstruction but skin, fascia or muscle can be included in pedicled flaps.

MYOCUTANEOUS AND FASCIOCUTANEOUS FLAPS

Myocutaneous flaps consist of skin and the underlying muscle where the blood supply to the skin is derived from musculocutaneous perforating

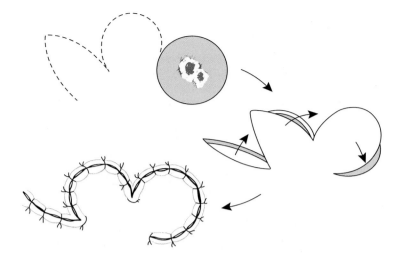

Fig. 14.4 Bilobed flap.

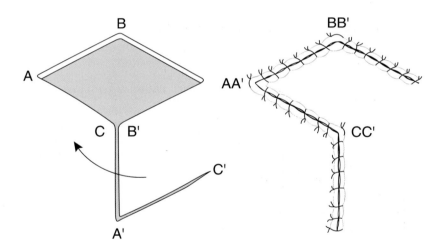

Fig. 14.5 Rhomboid flap.

vessels. All or part of the muscle can be transferred with a paddle of skin as a local, pedicled or free flap. Fasciocutaneous flaps rely on blood vessels that pass along the fibrous septa between muscle bellies or muscle compartments (septocutaneous perforators), and then spread out at the level of the deep fascia to form plexuses which in turn form branches to the skin (Fig. 14.6). These perforating blood vessels enhance the surviving length-to-width ratio of these flaps especially in the reconstruction of defects of the lower limb.

Free flaps
Any tissue that can be isolated on a vascular pedicle can be transferred as a free flap using microvascular anastomoses to a distant site with success rates of

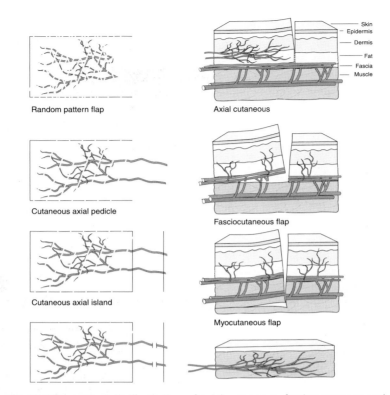

Fig. 14.6 Diagrammatic illustration of axial cutaneous, fasciocutaneous and myocutaneous flaps.

95%. Free flaps have many advantages over conventional flaps. These include the freedom to tailor exactly the requirements of the defect in terms of the size and tissue required (skin, fascia, muscle, bone or combination) without the constraints of a pedicle. There is a wide choice of donor sites that allows the use of an appropriate flap which produces a minimum donor defect.

Key points for clinical practice

- Skin lesions of doubtful aetiology should be subject to a punch or small incision biopsy except where a melanoma is suspected.

- Excision margins are then dictated by the size and type of skin carcinoma.

- All suspected melanomas should be biopsied by excision. Incision biopsies interfere with accurate Breslow thickness determination which guides ultimate excision margins of melanoma.

- If direct closure is not possible, reconstruction is carried out using either skin grafts or flaps.

- The choice of reconstructive procedure should be guided by the size of defect, type of tissue required as well as functional and aesthetic considerations.

References

1. Wade TR, Ackerman AB. The many faces of basal cell carcinoma. J Dermatol Surg Oncol 1978; 23: 23.
2. Dubin N, Kopf AW. Multivariate risk score for recurrence of cutaneous basal cell carcinomas. Arch Dermatol 1983; 119: 373.
3. Epstein E. How accurate is the visual assessment of basal cell carcinomas. Br J Dermatol 1973; 89: 37.
4. Wolf DJ, Zitelli JA. Surgical margins for BCC. Arch Dermatol 1987; 123: 340.
5. Sexton M, Jones DB, Maloney ME. Histologic pattern analysis of basal cell carcinoma. J Am Acad Dermatol 1990; 23: 1118.
6. Cottel WI, Proper S. Mohs' surgery, fresh-tissue techniques. Our technique with a review. J Dermatol Surg Oncol 1982; 8: 576.
7. Salasche SJ. Curettage and electrodessication in the treatment of midfacial basal cell epithelioma. J Am Acad Dermatol 1983; 8: 496.
8. Zacarian SA. Cryosurgery of cutaneous carcinomas. An 18 year study of 3022 patients with 4,228 carcinomas. J Am Acad Dermatol 1983; 9: 947.
9. Bandieramonte G, Lepera P, Moglia D et al. Laser microsurgery for superficial T1-T2 basal cell carcinoma of the eyelid margins. Ophthalmology 1997; 104: 1179. 10. Humphreys TR, Malhotra R, Scharf MJ et al. Treatment of superficial basal cell carcinoma and squamous cell carcinoma in situ with a high-energy pulsed carbon-dioxide. Arch Dermatol 1998; 134: 1247.
11. Hauben DJ. The biologic behaviour of basal cell carcinoma, Part I. Plast Reconstr Surg 1982; 69: 103.
12. Hauben DJ. The biologic behaviour of basal cell carcinoma, Part II. Plast Reconstr Surg 1982; 69: 110.
13. Hayes H. Basal cell carcinoma: The East Grinstead Experience. Plast Reconstr Surg 1962; 30: 273.
14. Taylor GA, Barrisoni D. Ten year's experience in the surgical treatment of basal cell carcinoma. Br J Surg 1973; 60: 522.
15. Pascal RR. Prognosis of 'incompletely excised' versus 'completely excised' basal cell carcinoma. Plast Reconstr Surg 1968; 41: 328.
16. Sussman LA, Liggins DF. Incompletely excised basal cell carcinoma: a management dilemma? Aust N Z J Surg 1996; 66: 276.
17. Rowe DE, Carroll CL, Day CL. Long term recurrence rates in previously treated (primary) basal cell carcinoma: implications for patient follow up. J Dermatol Surg Oncol 1989; 15: 315.
18. Koplin L, Zarem HA. Recurrent basal cell carcinoma. A review concerning the incidence, behaviour, and management of recurrent basal cell carcinoma, with emphasis on the incompletely excised lesion. Plast Reconstr Surg 1980; 65: 656.
19. Luce EA. Oncologic considerations in non-melanotic skin cancer. Clin Plast Surg 1995; 22: 39.
20. Brodland DG, Zitelli GA. Surgical margins for excision of primary cutaneous squamous cell carcinoma. J Am Acad Dermatol 1992; 27: 108.
21. Roth JJ, Granick MS. Squamous cell and adnexal carcinomas of the skin. Clin Plast Surg 1997; 24: 687.
22. Lawrence N, Cottel WI. Squamous cell carcinoma of skin with perineural invasion. J Am Acad Dermatol 1994; 31: 1994.
23. Mohs FE. Chemosurgery. Clin Plast Surg 1980; 7: 349.
24. Rowe DE, Carrol RJ, Day CL. Prognostic factors for local recurrence, metastasis, and survival rates in squamous cell carcinoma of the skin, ear, and lip: implications for treatment modality selection. J Am Acad Dermatol 1992; 26: 976.
25. North JH, Spellman JE, Driscoll D et al. Advanced cutaneous squamous cell carcinoma of the trunk and extremity: analysis of prognostic factors. J Surg Oncol 1997; 64: 212.
26. Breslow A, Macht SD. Optimal size of resection margin for thin cutaneous melanoma. Surg Gynecol Obstet 1977; 145: 691–692.
27. Veronesi U, Cascinelli N, Adamus J et al. Thin stage I primary cutaneous malignant melanoma. Comparison of excision with margins of 1 or 3 cm [published erratum appears in N Engl J Med 1991; 325: 292]. N Engl J Med 1988; 318: 1159–1162.

28. Veronesi U, Cascinelli N. Narrow excision (1-cm margin). A safe procedure for thin cutaneous melanoma. Arch Surg 1991; 126: 438–441.

29. Balch CM, Urist MM, Karakousis CP et al. Efficacy of 2-cm surgical margins for intermediate-thickness melanomas (1 to 4 mm). Results of a multi-institutional randomized surgical trial [see comments]. Ann Surg 1993; 218: 262–267.

30. Harris MN, Shapiro RL, Roses DF. Malignant melanoma. Primary surgical management (excision and node dissection) based on pathology and staging [see comments]. Cancer 1995; 75 (Suppl. 2): 715–725.

31. Eva-Singletary S, Balch CM, Urist MM et al. Surgical treatment of primary melanoma. In: Balch CM. (ed) Cutaneous Melanoma. Philadelphia, PA: Lippincott, 1992: 269–274.

32. Beitsch P, Balch C. Operative morbidity and risk factor assessment in melanoma patients undergoing inguinal lymph node dissection. Am J Surg 1992; 164: 462–465.

33. Kissin MW, Simpson DA, Easton D, White H, Westbury G. Prognostic factors related to survival and groin recurrence following therapeutic lymph node dissection for lower limb malignant melanoma. Br J Surg 1987; 74: 1023–1026.

34. Milton GW, Shaw HM, McCarthy WH, Pearson L, Balch CM, Soong SJ. Prophylactic lymph node dissection in clinical stage I cutaneous malignant melanoma: results of surgical treatment in 1319 patients. Br J Surg 1982; 69: 108–111.

35. Reintgen DS, Cox EB, McCarty Jr KS, Vollmer RT, Seigler HF. Efficacy of elective lymph node dissection in patients with intermediate thickness primary melanoma. Ann Surg 1983; 198: 379–385.

36. Veronesi U, Adamus J, Bandiera DC et al. Inefficacy of immediate node dissection in stage 1 melanoma of the limbs. N Engl J Med 1977; 297: 627–630.

37. Sim FH, Taylor WF, Pritchard DJ, Soule EH. Lymphadenectomy in the management of stage I malignant melanoma: a prospective randomized study. Mayo Clin Proc 1986; 61: 697–705.

38. Cochran AJ, Wen DR, Morton DL. Management of the regional lymph nodes in patients with cutaneous malignant melanoma. World J Surg 1992; 16: 214–221.

39. Morton DL, Wen DR, Wong JH et al. Technical details of intraoperative lymphatic mapping for early stage melanoma. Arch Surg 1992; 127: 392–399.

40. Morton DL, Wanek L, Nizze JA, Elashoff RM, Wong JH. Improved long-term survival after lymphadenectomy of melanoma metastatic to regional nodes. Analysis of prognostic factors in 1134 patients from the John Wayne Cancer Clinic. Ann Surg 1991; 214: 491–499.

41. Chana JS, Fenton O. Tissue expansion. Recent Adv Surg 1997; 20: 203.

Alastair G.W. Moses   Kenneth C.H. Fearon

Cancer cachexia

Cachexia derives from the Greek *kakos*, meaning bad, and *hexis* condition. While cachexia may be found in patients with debilitating diseases such as chronic obstructive pulmonary disease, rheumatoid arthritis , cardiac failure and AIDS, its most frequent association is with advanced cancer. Often used to describe severe weight loss, the word cachexia represents a complex, multifactorial syndrome in which some or all of the following symptoms may be exhibited: anorexia, early satiety, hypophagia, fatigue, anaemia, oedema, and weight loss (characterised by excessive lean tissue wasting compared with undernutrition in an otherwise healthy individual). These symptoms combine to cause a reduction in mobility and quality of life and may even contribute to mortality.

OVERVIEW

Advanced cancer tends to be associated with anorexia and a reduction in food intake. The normal response to semistarvation is a reduction in energy expenditure and a fall in protein turnover such that energy and nitrogen stores are preserved. However, in the cancer patient this adaptive response is abnormal and whilst energy intake is decreased, basal energy expenditure is often increased and is accompanied by a negative nitrogen balance. Visceral protein mass is preserved at the expense of muscle tissue, and there is extensive loss of adipose tissue. The skeletal muscle loss may be of particular significance in the decreased quality of life and reduced functional ability recorded in cachectic patients.

At the centre of the cachectic process is the host–tumour relationship and the catabolic effects of conventional anti-neoplastic therapy. As a consequence

Mr Alastair G.W. Moses BSc FRCS, Clinical Research Fellow, Department of Clinical and Surgical Sciences (Surgery), Edinburgh Royal Infirmary, Lauriston Place, Edinburgh EH3 9YW, UK
Prof. Kenneth C.H. Fearon MD FRCS, Professor of Surgical Oncology and Honorary Consultant Surgeon, Department of Clinical and Surgical Sciences (Surgery), Edinburgh Royal Infirmary, Lauriston Place, Edinburgh EH3 9YW, UK (for correspondence)

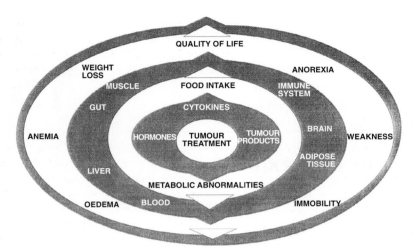

Fig. 15.1 The syndrome of cancer cachexia is a complex multilayered phenomenon. As a result of progressive tumour growth, a complex mixture of mediators are released. In turn, alterations in food intake and body metabolism result in loss of tissue/organ mass and function. Finally, these changes are experienced as a variety of symptoms and signs.

of these interactions, anorectic and catabolic mediators are released. Soluble pro-inflammatory cytokines (from the immune system and perhaps cancer cells), tumour-derived cachectic factors, and an alteration of the hormonal environment in favour of the counter-regulatory stress hormones causes a reduction in food intake and a series of changes in whole body metabolism. The function/mass of various organs and tissues is subsequently compromised leading to the symptoms and signs of cachexia (Fig. 15.1).

Simple hyperalimentation has not proved to be an effective therapy for cancer cachexia, presumably due to the underlying shift towards catabolic processes in the cachectic patient. Newer approaches need to focus on modulating the underlying metabolic abnormalities in order to allow appropriate utilisation of conventional nutritional support.

PREVALENCE

Without a unified definition there is little clear data on the prevalence of cachexia. However, most patients with advanced cancer will have lost weight and exhibit some of the other features of cachexia. Cancer of the lung and upper gastro-intestinal tract is particularly associated with wasting. However, within the same tumour type there may be marked inter-patient variation pointing to significant variations in tumour phenotype or patient genotype and the complexities of the tumour–host relationship which develops during disease progression.

IMPORTANCE OF CANCER CACHEXIA

SURVIVAL

In 1932, an autopsy study of 500 cancer patients found 22% had died primarily as a result of cachexia.[1] More recent studies have suggested the figure lies between 1–10%, with infection being the single most important cause of mortality in cancer patients.[2,3] However, malnutrition may be associated with a greater propensity to, and inability to fight, infection, and is thus likely still to be a major contributor to morbidity and mortality. Both the presence and degree of weight loss have been shown to relate to survival duration in patients with advanced cancer.[4,5]

OUTCOME FOLLOWING SURGERY

For patients with oesophageal and colorectal cancer, pre-operative weight loss of greater than 15% and 20%, respectively, has been associated with increased postoperative morbidity and mortality.[6,7] More recently, Hill and co-workers have shown that in patients undergoing major gastrointestinal surgery, protein depletion is associated with weaker respiratory muscles, greater risk of postoperative pneumonia, and longer hospital stay.[8] Weight loss greater than 10% was a less sensitive index and had to be accompanied by clinically obvious physiological impairment (such as reduced cough strength) before it was associated with increased postoperative complications.[9] Thus, with modern surgery and anaesthesia, early cachexia is certainly not a barrier to appropriate operative intervention.

QUALITY OF LIFE

In patients with advanced cancer, quality as well as quantity of life is important. Weight loss has been shown to be associated with decreased quality of life as well as performance scores in cancer patients.[10] Domains particularly affected include physical scores and mobility, probably as a result of muscle wasting. However, symptoms such as anorexia or nausea can also be very unpleasant for patients. Hence improvement or even stabilisation of quality of life is now a valid end-point for intervention. Furthermore, quality of life assessment is now almost mandatory in any clinical trial involving patients with cancer.

MECHANISMS OF CACHEXIA

Weight loss due to inadequate nutrient intake is a key feature of cachexia. Quantitatively inadequate caloric intake is the greatest contributor to patients' negative energy balance.

Key points 1–4

In cancer patients:

- Increasing severity of weight loss is associated with reduced survival.
- Loss of 20% of pre-illness weight is associated with increased surgical mortality.
- 10% weight loss with physiological impairment increases surgical complications.
- Weight loss is associated with decreased quality of life.

ANOREXIA

Loss of appetite is a frequent symptom in advanced cancer. The causes of anorexia are multifactorial, and can be divided into those related directly to the disease and its treatment, and those occurring as part of the cachexia syndrome (Table 15.1).

Disease-related factors include: partial or complete gastrointestinal obstruction, nausea, constipation, malabsorption, obstructive jaundice, debility, pain, anxiety, depression, and iatrogenic factors such as recent surgery, opiates, and radio- or chemotherapy. Active treatment of these problems is mandatory if optimal food intake is to be achieved. However, even when these factors have been dealt with successfully, many patients will still have a background of persistent anorexia which is independent of physical factors and appears to be intimately related to the cachexia syndrome.

In otherwise healthy humans, under-nutrition and weight loss are potent stimuli of increased appetite. That anorexia persists in cancer cachexia implies a block in the normal feedback mechanisms governing appetite. Recent studies in rodents have provided a strong body of evidence regarding the regulation of normal feeding behaviour and have provided possible mechanisms to account for the anorexia observed in cancer cachexia.

Energy homeostasis is regulated in the hypothalamus, where production of neuropeptide Y (NPY) leads to an increase in appetite and, on the other hand, production of CRF causes a decrease in appetite. It has been suggested that in cachexia, as in sepsis, pro-inflammatory cytokines are responsible for many of the underlying metabolic disturbances. These cytokines such as tumour necrosis factor alpha (TNF-α) and particularly interleukin 1 (IL-1), can act either directly after crossing the blood–brain barrier, or indirectly via the vagus nerve to inhibit the production or action of NPY. Other antagonists of NPY such as central levels of serotonin and corticotropin releasing factor (CRF) may also be influenced by IL-1.[11]

It has been suggested that leptin, an adipocyte-derived hormone which induces anorexia and hypermetabolism at the hypothalamic level in response to fat deposition, could be involved in the anorexia of cachexia. However, initial studies have suggested leptin levels are low (although appropriate for the reduced body adiposity found in patients with cancer cachexia) and certainly not elevated.[12] It remains possible that leptin may have a more subtle influence on cancer anorexia.

EARLY SATIETY

Even when cancer patients do feel hungry, they often experience symptoms of fullness and bloating after eating very small quantities of food. This early

Table 15.1 Causes of anorexia in cancer patients

* Gastrointestinal tract obstruction	* Pain
* Nausea	* Anxiety
* Constipation	* Depression
* Malabsorption	* Tumour-mediated effects
* Obstructive jaundice	
* Treatment (including opiates, recent surgery, radiotherapy and chemotherapy)	

satiety is due to delayed gastric emptying, and can significantly diminish caloric intake.

One of the main peripheral satiety factors appears to be cholecystokinin (CCK), a peptide produced in the duodenal wall which stimulates afferent vagal fibres. Again cytokines such as IL-1 appear to stimulate CCK and decrease gastric transit.[11] Thus the inflammatory response that occurs in some advanced cancer patients may be important in the aetiology of early satiety.

HYPERMETABOLISM

Over the long-term, hypermetabolism may be a contributing factor to negative energy balance, and weight loss. Patients with tumour types associated with cachexia such as lung and upper gastrointestinal cancer are often hypermetabolic. However, even in individuals with the same neoplasm, wide variations in basal metabolism have been reported (varying from 60–150% of predicted values).[13] Furthermore, it is now recognised that during the development of cachexia patients may progress from a hypermetabolic to a hypometabolic state.

SUBSTRATE METABOLISM

Carbohydrate metabolism

Human tumours metabolise glucose anaerobically to lactate. Overall, glucose turnover is increased in cancer cachexia with peripheral tissues exhibiting insulin resistance. The energy-dependant Cori cycle is up-regulated in the liver (converting lactate back to glucose[21]).[14] The peripheral insulin resistance observed in cachexia is probably a major factor contributing to the suboptimal response to nutritional support in cancer patients.

Lipid metabolism

While excessive lean tissue loss differentiates cachexia from simple starvation, reduced fat mass accounts for the greatest loss of body weight.[15] Decreased lipogenesis with normal lipolysis has been noted to occur.[16] Whether this is part of the cachectic process or merely adaptive to energy deprivation is not clear. A variety of lipid mobilising factors have been identified in certain animal models of cachexia.

Protein metabolism

Protein turnover is generally increased in cachectic cancer patients.[17] The mobilisation of amino acids from peripheral tissues such as skeletal muscle may be partly to provide key amino acids which are required for increased visceral protein synthesis, e.g. acute phase proteins.

THE ACUTE PHASE PROTEIN RESPONSE

The acute phase protein response (APPR) is a stereotypical phenomenon found in patients subjected to major trauma, surgical insult or sepsis. During the acute phase response, positive acute phase reactants such as fibrinogen and C-reactive protein are exported in increased quantities by the liver and serve in the processes of healing and repair. However, the APPR is also found in patients with cancer cachexia, and is particularly associated with tumours of the pancreas, lung, oesophagus and kidney. In the chronic situation, the APPR may no longer be advantageous and may simply lead to the accelerated loss of lean tissue. Indeed, the presence of such a response has been shown to be associated with accelerated weight loss and decreased survival in several tumour types, and in pancreatic cancer has been reported to increase in severity with disease progression.[18]

MEDIATORS OF CACHEXIA

Traditionally, cachexia was thought to result directly from tumour parasitism. However, profound wasting can occur in association with very small neoplasms. Thus, cachexia cannot result simply from the cancer feeding on all available nutrients at the expense of its host. Rodent studies demonstrate cachexia is mediated by circulating factors derived either from the tumour directly or from the host in response to the tumour.[19]

CYTOKINES

Pro-inflammatory cytokines such as IL-1, TNF-α, interferon gamma (IFN-γ), and IL-6 appear to underlie many of the abnormal metabolic manifestations of cachexia. These are produced by activated white blood cells, although there is some evidence from tumour cell lines that cancer cells can also release them.

NEUROTRANSMITTERS

As has been mentioned previously with regard to anorexia, animal studies suggest dysregulation of hypothalamic neuropeptidergic pathways involving the neurotransmitters NPY, CRF and serotonin may lead to the development of cancer-related anorexia. In turn, these may be regulated by pro-inflammatory cytokines (see above).

HORMONES

Serum cortisol levels are increased in cachectic cancer patients. In contrast, insulin levels are decreased and peripheral insulin resistance is increased. A shift in the insulin/cortisol ratio in favour of cortisol may help to explain the trend towards catabolism.[20]

TUMOUR-SPECIFIC PRODUCTS

A glycoprotein, proteolysis inducing factor (PIF), has recently been shown to cause muscle wasting in a murine cancer cachexia model and has also been isolated from the urine of weight losing cancer patients.[21] PIF is produced by tumour cell lines, and it may be that in vivo this tumour-derived product is partially responsible for the significant muscle wasting observed.

MANAGEMENT OF CANCER CACHEXIA

The best treatment for cancer cachexia is to cure the cancer. However, the majority of patients with cachexia have tumours that are too advanced at diagnosis for

> **Key point 5**
>
> - It is important to take a holistic approach to the overall care of patients with cancer cachexia.

this to be possible. In these patients, it is important to take a holistic approach to their overall care and define areas which require attention (Table 15.2). Two issues which require further discussion are the merits of nutritional intervention, and pharmacological approaches to the treatment of cachexia.

NUTRITIONAL INTERVENTION

The cachectic patient undergoing surgery

Over the past 20 years, a multitude of studies have looked at the potential benefits of peri-operative nutrition in cancer patients undergoing major surgery. Unlike nutrition for multiple trauma or severe burns patients, the place of nutritional intervention in cancer patients remains controversial both for enteral and parenteral routes of administration.

The majority of studies have not demonstrated significant advantages associated with peri-operative nutrition in cancer patients.[22,23] Particularly in the case of parenteral nutrition, net harm may be associated with the intervention (specifically line-related complications such as catheter sepsis). However, most cancer patients undergoing surgery have potentially resectable tumours and have not suffered significant wasting prior to their operation. The question, therefore, remains unanswered: if a cancer patient with severe malnutrition is to undergo elective or emergency surgery, will they benefit from peri-operative nutritional support? There is certainly no doubt that these patients have a far higher risk of complications and death. However, difficulties encountered in recruiting enough of these patients into any one trial makes answering the above question problematic.

The one study often quoted as addressing the above issue randomised 459 patients (of whom 66% had cancer) to receive either peri-operative TPN or no nutritional support in association with major surgical procedures.[24] Within a small subgroup analysis of severely malnourished patients, there was no difference in infectious complications, while the TPN fed group had less non-

Table 15.2 Clinical management of cachexia

- Correct factors which may contribute to reduced food intake (e.g. pain)
- Correct factors contributing to debility (e.g. anaemia)
- Optimise food intake with appetising food, dietetic support, nutritional supplements
- Encourage mobility as endogenous anabolic stimulus
- Correct underlying metabolic abnormalities with anti-inflammatory agents such as NSAIDs or fish oil
- Use steroids/progestational agents to improve mood and appetite. Caution required due to potential side-effects.

> **Key point 6**
> - In cancer patients undergoing major surgery:
>   - Routine nutritional intervention is not efficacious.
>   - Severe malnutrition represents weight loss >15–20% of pre-illness level.
>   - Patients with severe malnutrition will probably benefit from nutritional support.
>   - The enteral route should be used wherever possible.

infectious and major complications. The difference between groups for major complications, while being numerically large, was not statistically significant, perhaps due to inadequate sample size.

Nutritional support outwith surgery

The malnutrition associated with cancer cachexia is a chronic condition which has occurred over a period of months. Parenteral nutrition is costly, involves substantial patient education and may have an uncertain impact on quality of life if provided on a long-term basis. Moreover, significant complications such as catheter sepsis may be associated with this form of intervention. This led the American College of Physicians to publish a consensus document stating that in cancer patients 'parenteral nutritional support was associated with net harm, and no conditions could be defined in which such treatment appeared to be of benefit'.[25]

Two large studies have addressed oral nutritional supplementation in advanced cancer patients with a variety of malignancies undergoing palliative chemotherapy.[26,27] Patients were randomised to receive frequent nutritional counselling/nutritional supplements or to take an ad libitum diet. The counselled group increased significantly both their calorie and protein intake. However, there was no benefit in terms of weight, anthropometric measures, tumour response rate, survival or quality of life. Thus whilst all measures should be employed to decrease anorexia and enable cancer patients to maintain a reasonable nutritional intake, there is no evidence to suggest that aggressive conventional nutritional intervention in terms of TPN or EN is justified. These findings emphasise that the cancer cachexia syndrome is not merely related to under nutrition, but metabolic changes have occurred which restrict anabolism even when extra calories and protein can be supplied.

PHARMACOLOGICAL APPROACHES

The failure of conventional nutritional support to alter the progressive wasting associated with cachexia has prompted the search for pharmacological agents

> **Key point 7**
> - Standard nutritional support will not reverse cancer cachexia.

Table 15.3 Benefits and limitations of pharmaceuticals used in cachexia

Steroids	Improve mood and appetite Side effects preclude long-term use
Non-steroidal anti-inflammatory drugs	May slow weight-loss and improve survival Caution required due to potential for GI bleeding effects
Progestational agents	Improve appetite. Cause fluid retention
Fish oil	Appears to stabilise weight and may prolong survival. Generally non-toxic

which may modulate the underlying metabolic dysfunction which promotes catabolism at the expense of anabolism (Table 15.3).

Corticosteroids

Corticosteroids are used frequently by palliative care physicians to improve appetite, reduce nausea and create a psychological sense of well-being. Their potential efficacy in cancer-related cachexia has been well scrutinised. Both prednisolone (15 mg/day) and dexamethasone (3–6 mg/day) have been shown to improve appetite versus placebo. Indeed intravenous methylprednisolone (125 mg/day) has been suggested to increase quality of life.[28] However, corticosteroids have not been shown to halt tissue wasting, and their beneficial effects are relatively short-lived. Furthermore, unwanted side-effects include: fluid retention, muscle breakdown and insulin resistance. As such steroids tend to be reserved for therapy during the preterminal phase of a patient's illness.

Non-steroidal anti-inflammatory drugs

In cachectic cancer patients, the non-steroidal anti-inflammatory drug ibuprofen has been shown to reduce serum levels of IL-6, cortisol, and acute phase proteins and to reduce abnormally elevated whole body protein turnover.[29,30] Ibuprofen will also reduce elevated resting energy expenditure and acute phase proteins in pancreatic cancer patients.[31] When either prednisolone or indomethacin were administered to a heterogeneous group of advanced cancer patients, survival was increased when compared with placebo.[32] Concerns remain regarding potential gastrointestinal haemorrhage in debilitated individuals treated with these medications. The use of Cox-2 inhibitors may obviate this problem. However, the efficacy of non-steroidal drugs combined with conventional nutritional support remains to be tested in a prospective manner.

Progestational agents

Following the observation of unexpected weight gain associated with megestrol acetate therapy in advanced breast cancer, there has been much interest in the potential anti-cachectic effects of such progestational agents. A number of randomised trials in heterogeneous groups of advanced cancer patients have demonstrated improved appetite and weight stabilisation.[33] The mechanism of action of appetite improvement is unknown, but may be related to a reduction in pro-inflammatory cytokine production. However, most of the weight gain with these compounds may be due to fluid retention or fat deposition with little effect on lean tissue. As well as peripheral oedema, these agents are associated with an increased risk of venous thrombo-embolism and, more worryingly, a recent trial of megestrol acetate in patients receiving chemotherapy demonstrated a poorer tumour response and trend towards decreased survival in the treatment group.[34] These drugs, therefore, may be beneficial as appetite stimulants, but care must be taken with unwanted side-effects. Again their use is generally recommended for patients in a preterminal phase.

Omega-3 fatty acids

Recent evidence has suggested eicosapentanoic acid (EPA), an essential polyunsaturated fatty acid found in high concentrations in 'oily' fish, may be a putative anti-cachectic agent. EPA appears to have two separate potential modes of activity: on the one hand down-regulation of pro-inflammatory cytokines and the acute phase response, and on the other acting directly on tumour cells to prevent the release of tumour-derived anti cachectic factors, perhaps causing tumour cell death via apoptosis. Uncontrolled studies with fish oil and pure EPA capsules (2–6 g EPA) have demonstrated weight stability in previously weight losing pancreatic cancer patients.[35,36] A randomised study of fish oil capsules and vitamin E in advanced cancer patients has demonstrated a significantly longer survival compared with the placebo group.[37]

Key point 8

- The benefits and limitations of pharmaceuticals used in cachexia are show in Table 15.3.

COMBINED NUTRITIONAL AND PHARMACOLOGICAL APPROACHES

Great interest has been generated over the past few years in 'neutraceuticals'; clinical nutrition supplements enriched with compounds capable of modulating immune function or suppressing exuberant inflammatory responses in patients subjected in particular to trauma or surgical stress. For the treatment of cancer cachexia, the idea of suppressing the pro-inflammatory response and damping down catabolic processes while at the same time supplying extra calories and protein which could be incorporated into lean tissue is an attractive one. In a study designed to test this, 20 weight-losing pancreatic cancer patients received fish oil enriched oral nutritional supplements (providing 2 g EPA, 600 kcal and 30 g protein/day).[38] Weight loss

---

Key point 9

- The future of anti-cachectic treatment lies in normalising catabolic processes while providing nutritional intervention.

Key points for clinical practice

In cancer patients:

- The degree of weight loss is associated with reduced survival.
- Loss of 20% of pre-illness weight is associated with increased surgical mortality.
- 10% weight loss with physiological impairment increases surgical complications.
- Weight loss is associated with decreased quality of life.
- It is important to take a holistic approach to the overall care of patients with cancer cachexia (Table 15.2).
- In cancer patients undergoing major surgery:

  Routine nutritional intervention is not efficacious.

  Severe malnutrition represents weight loss >15–20% of pre-illness level.

  Patients with severe malnutrition will probably benefit from nutritional support.

  The enteral route should be used wherever possible
- Standard nutritional support will not reverse cancer cachexia.
- There are benefits and limitations to the use of pharmaceutical agents in cachexia: see Table 15.3.
- The future of anti-cachectic treatment lies in normalising catabolic processes whilst providing what would be considered conventional nutritional support.

was reversed, and appetite and performance status were improved. Very significantly, the weight gain was accompanied by accretion of lean tissue, implying that as a result of consuming the sip feed, anabolic signals were able to predominate over catabolic ones. The results of a randomised trial are now awaited.

References

1. Warren S. The immediate causes of death in cancer. Am J Med Sci 1935; 184: 610–616.
2. Inagaki J, Rodriguez V, Bodey GP. Causes of death in cancer patients. Cancer 1974; 33: 568–573.
3. Ambrus JL, Ambrus CM, Mink IB, Pickren JW. Causes of death in cancer patients. J Med 1975; 6: 61–64.
4. DeWys WD, Begg C, Lavin PT et al. Prognostic effect of weight loss prior to chemotherapy in cancer patients. Am J Med 1980; 69: 491–497.
5. Falconer JS, Fearon KCH, Ross JA et al. Acute-phase protein response and survival duration of patients with pancreatic cancer. Cancer 1995; 75: 2077–2082.
6. Conti S, West JP, Fitzpatrick HF. Mortality and morbidity after esophagogastrectomy for cancer of the esophagus and cardia. Am Surg 1977; 43: 92–96.

7. Hickman DM, Miller RA, Rombeau JL, Twomey PL, Frey CF. Serum albumin and body weight as predictors of postoperative course in colorectal cancer. JPEN 1980; 4: 314–316.

8. Windsor JA, Hill GL. Risk factors for postoperative pneumonia. The importance of protein depletion. Ann Surg 1988; 208: 209–214.

9. Windsor JA, Hill GL. Weight loss with physiologic impairment. A basic indicator of surgical risk. Ann Surg 1988; 207: 290–296.

10. O'Gorman P, McMillan DC, McArdle CS. Impact of weight loss, appetite, and the inflammatory response on quality of life in gastrointestinal cancer patients. Nut Cancer 1998; 32: 76–80..

11. Inui A. Cancer anorexia-cachexia syndrome: are neuropeptides the key? Cancer Res 1999; 59: 3393–4501.

12. Wallace AM, Sattar N, McMillan DC. Effect of weight loss and the inflammatory response on leptin concentration in gastrointestinal cancer patients. Clin Cancer Res 1998; 2977–2979.

13. Knox LS, Crosby LO, Feurer ID et al. Energy expenditure in malnourished cancer patients. Ann Surg 1983; 197: 152–162.

14. Edén E, Edström S, Bennegård K et al. Glucose flux in relation to energy expenditure in malnourished patients with and without cancer during periods of fasting and feeding. Cancer Res 1984; 44: 1718–1724.

15. Fearon KCH, Preston T. Body composition in cancer cachexia. Infusionstherapie 1990; 17 (Suppl. 3): 63–66.

16. Jeevanandam M, Horowitz GD, Lowry SF et al. Cancer cachexia and the rate of whole body lipolysis in man. Metabolism 1986; 35: 304–310

17. Fearon KCH, Hansell DT, Preston P et al. Influence of whole body protein turnover rate on resting energy expenditure in patients with cancer. Cancer Res 1988; 48: 2590–2595.

18. Falconer JS, Fearon KCH, Plester CE et al. Cytokines, the acute-phase response, and resting energy expenditure in cachectic patients with pancreatic cancer. Ann Surg 1994; 219: 325–331.

19. Norton JA, Moley JF, Green MV et al. Parabiotic transfer of cancer anorexia/cachexia in male rats. Cancer Res 1985; 45: 5547–5552.

20. Fearon KCH, Falconer JS, Slater C et al. Albumin synthesis rates are not decreased in hypoalbuminaemic cachectic cancer patients with an ongoing acute phase response. Ann Surg 1998; 227: 249–254.

21. Todorov P, Cariuk P, McDevitt T et al. Characterisation of a cancer cachectic factor. Nature 1996; 379: 739–742.

22. Heyland DK, MacDonald S, Laurie RD, Drover JW. Total parenteral nutrition in the critically ill patient: a meta-analysis. JAMA 1998; 280: 2013–2019.

23. Silk DBA, Green CJ. Perioperative nutrition: parenteral versus enteral. Curr Opin Clin Nutr Met Care 1998; 1: 21–27.

24. The Veterans Affairs Total Parenteral Nutrition Co-operative Study Group. Perioperative total parenteral nutrition in surgical patients. N Engl J Med 1991; 325: 525–532.

25. American College of Physicians. Parenteral nutrition in patients receiving cancer chemotherapy. Ann Intern Med 1989; 110: 734–736.

26. Evans WK, Nixon DW, Daly JM et al. A randomised trial of oral nutritional support versus ad lib nutritional intake during chemotherapy for advanced colorectal and non-small-cell lung cancer. J Clin Oncol 5: 1987; 113–124.

27. Ovesen L, Hannibal J, Mortensen EL. The interrelationship of weight loss, dietary intake, and quality of life in ambulatory patients with cancer of the lung, breast, and ovary. Nutr Cancer 1993; 19: 159–167.

28. Gagnon B, Bruera E. A review of the drug treatment of cachexia associated with cancer. Drugs 1998; 55: 675–688.

29. McMillan DC, Leen E, Smith J et al. Effect of extended ibuprofen administration on the acute phase protein response in colorectal cancer patients. Eur J Surg Oncol 1995; 21: 531–534.

30. Preston T, Fearon KCH, McMillan DC et al. Effect of ibuprofen on the acute-phase response and protein metabolism in patients with cancer and weight loss. Br J Surg 1995; 82: 229–234.

31. Wigmore SJ, Falconer JS, Plester CE et al. Ibuprofen reduces energy expenditure and acute-phase protein production compared with placebo in pancreatic cancer patients. Br J Cancer 1995; 72: 185–188.

32. Lundholm K, Gelin J, Hyltander A et al. Anti-inflammatory treatment may prolong survival in undernourished patients with metastatic solid tumours. Cancer Res 1994; 54: 5602–5606.

33. Ottery FD, Walsh D, Strawford A. Pharmacologic management of anorexia/cachexia. Semin Oncol 1998; 25: (Suppl. 6): 35–44.

34. Rowland KM, Loprinzi CL, Shaw EG et al. Randomised double-blind placebo-controlled trial of cisplatin and etoposide plus megestrol acetate/placebo in extensive-stage small-cell lung cancer: A North Central Cancer Treatment Group Study. J Clin Oncol 1996; 14: 135–141.

35. Wigmore SJ, Ross JA, Falconer JS et al. The effect of polyunsaturated fatty acids on the progress of cachexia in patients with pancreatic cancer. Nutrition 1996; 12 (Suppl): S27–S30.

36. Wigmore SJ, Barber MD, Ross JA, Tisdale MJ, Fearon KCH. The effect of oral eicosapentaenoic acid on weight loss in patients with pancreatic cancer. Nutr Cancer 2000; 36: 177–184.

37. Gogos CA, Ginopoulos P, Salsa B et al. Dietary omega-3 polyunsaturated fatty acids plus vitamin E restore immunodeficiency and prolong survival for severely ill patients with generalised malignancy: a randomised controlled trial. Cancer 1998; 82: 395–402.

38. Barber MD, Ross JA, Voss AC et al. The effect of an oral nutritional supplement enriched with fish oil on weight-loss in patients with pancreatic cancer. Br J Cancer 1999; 81:80–86.

Bryony E. Lovett   I. Taylor

Recent randomised controlled trials in general surgery

Historically, less than 10% of published articles in general surgery are in the form of randomised controlled trials. In a departure from previous practice, this chapter outlines a number of randomised trials, of interest to surgeons, published during 1999 and 2000.

GENERAL SURGERY

HERNIA REPAIR

The MRC Laparoscopic Groin Hernia Trial[1] compared laparoscopic and open hernia repair in 928 patients. At 1 week, 29.9% of laparoscopic and 43.5% of open patients had at least one complication (95% CI -20.6% to -6.6% $P < 0.001$). The laparoscopic group returned to normal social activity significantly earlier than the open group and at 1 year had a lower rate of persistent groin pain. However, all seven recurrences occurred in the laparoscopic group (1.9% versus 0% [95% CI for difference 0.5–3.4%], $P = 0.017$). A number of other trials comparing laparoscopic and open repair have concluded that the laparoscopic repair facilitates earlier return to work, with less postoperative pain but at greater expense and with higher complication rates.[2–4]

The Shouldice technique is historically recognised as the gold standard for hernia repair. The Lichtenstein tension free mesh technique has become increasingly popular and is easily taught. Danielson compared these procedures in 178 patients operated upon by trainees.[5] Duration of operation and complication rates were similar. Mesh repair resulted in less days of sick leave (18 versus 23 days, $P < 0.05$) and fewer recurrences (nil versus 9 days, $P <0.01$).

Miss Bryony E. Lovett MChir FRCS, Lecturer, Department of Surgery, University College London, Charles Bell House, 67–73 Riding House Street, London W1P 7LD, UK (for correspondence)
Prof. I. Taylor MD ChM FRCS, Professor and Head, Department of Surgery, University College London, Charles Bell House, 67–73 Riding House Street, London W1P 7LD, UK

LAPAROSCOPIC SURGERY

Postoperative nausea and vomiting (PONV) are responsible for considerable morbidity in up to 42% of patients after laparoscopic cholecystectomy. In a study comparing granisetron, droperidol and metoclopramide for PONV a high dose of granisetron (40 µg/kg) was the most effective.[6]

Bipolar electrocautery cutting forceps are equally efficacious to harmonic coagulating shears during the division of the short gastric vessels to facilitate gastric fundoplication. Intra-operative complications, gastric serosal burns and splenic capsule injury were equivalent in a trial of 86 patients.[7] Financial considerations favour the bipolar device.

TRANSFUSION

Traditionally, transfusion is given to patients if the haemoglobin (Hb) falls to below 10 g/dl. Hebert studied 838 patients admitted to ITU with Hb < 9 g/dl.[8] Those who were transfused only if the Hb fell further to < 7 g/dl had similar 30 day mortality to those immediately transfused, but their in-hospital mortality was 22.2% compared to 28.1% of the group whose transfusion was triggered by Hb <10 g/dl.

BREAST

SCREENING AND PREVENTION

Over 60,000 women have been included in the Edinburgh randomised trial of breast cancer screening.[9] Unadjusted results at 14 years showed a reduction in mortality of 13% which when adjusted for socio-economic status was 21%. This benefit extended to women under 50 years old.

Amongst postmenopausal women with osteoporosis taking raloxifene for 3 years, the relative risk of invasive breast cancer is reduced by 76%. Raloxifene reduced the risk of ER+ breast cancer by 90% (95% CI 0.04–0.24) but not ER− cancers in 7705 randomised women. Relative risk of DVT increased (RR = 3.1) without increased risk of endometrial cancer.[10]

ANTIBIOTIC PROPHYLAXIS

The efficacy of antibiotic prophylaxis in breast surgery using short (ceftazidime) and long (ceftriaxone) acting cephalosporins was evaluated in a trial of 1766 patients.[11] A single dose of 2 g of either antibiotic was given i.v. at induction. The patients who received ceftriaxone prophylaxis had 54.4% fewer overall infections than those who received ceftazidime prophylaxis. Wound infection occurred in 0.45% of the ceftriaxone recipients and 0.91% of the ceftazidime recipients (8 of 883).

CHEMOTHERAPY/RADIOTHERAPY

Hata et al.[12] have studied the effect of combination therapy with UFT (Tegafur; an anti-neoplastic agent which releases fluorouracil in vivo) and mitomycin plus tamoxifen as postoperative adjuvant therapy in the treatment of patients with stage II, oestrogen receptor positive (ER^+) primary breast cancer. On the day of surgery, mitomycin was administered intravenously at 13 mg/m^2. ER^+ patients were randomly allocated to either group A (n = 213), which received oral tamoxifen 20 mg/day, 14 days after surgery for 2 years, or group B (n = 223), receiving oral UFT 400 mg/day plus tamoxifen 20 mg/day. There was no significant difference in 5-year survival rates; however, relapse-free survival was 83.1% for group A and 90.7% for group B, a significant advantage (P = 0.020).

Interim results from the European Organization for Research and Treatment of Cancer (EORTC) Boost Versus No Boost trial[13] have evaluated the influence of a 16 Gy radiotherapy boost on the cosmetic outcome after 3 years of follow-up in patients treated with breast-conserving therapy. Results showed that a boost dose had a negative, but limited, impact on the cosmetic outcome after 3 years when assessed by a panel and by digitizer measurements.

Breast cancer patients treated with left-sided radiation therapy and doxorubicin (DOX) may have an increased risk of cardiac toxicity. The possible effects of different sequencing of radiotherapy and chemotherapy (CT) on cardiotoxicity, cellulitis, arm oedema, or brachial plexopathy, is poorly understood. In a trial of 244 patients with clinical stage I or II breast cancer treated with DOX of 180 mg/m^2 and radiotherapy, treatment to the left and right breast with initial chemotherapy or initial radiotherapy were compared.[14] Median follow-up time was 53 months. No cardiac events were observed for patients with either left- or right-sided breast cancer. The sequencing of chemotherapy and radiotherapy had no significant effect on the risk of cardiac toxicity, cellulitis, arm oedema or brachial plexopathy.

Mauriac et al.[15] published follow-up results from a trial of neo-adjuvant chemotherapy in the treatment of locally advanced breast disease. 272 patients with operable breast cancer > 3 cm diameter were randomised to receive initial mastectomy and axillary node dissection then chemotherapy or the same chemotherapy followed by surgery adjusted according to clinical response. At 34 months, patients who received initial chemotherapy suffered higher local recurrence but experienced better overall survival (P = 0.04). At median follow-up of 124 months, survival was identical in the two treatment groups, although breast conserving surgery was initially performed in 63%, after neo-adjuvant chemotherapy this rate had decreased to 45%.

In a comparison of CMF (cyclophosphamide, methotrexate and 5-fluorouracil) and MM (methotrexate and mitoxantrone) chemotherapy regimens for locally advanced or metastatic breast cancer in 116 patients, those receiving CMF had a significantly improved response (29% versus 15%, CI 1–19%, P < 0.07) but no significant differences in survival or quality of life were detected. Despite earlier relapse of disease, the MM regimen was associated with fewer side-effects and could still be considered as first line treatment in elderly or infirm patients.[16]

Patients with breast cancer and at least one lytic bone lesion were randomised to receive 90 mg pamidronate or placebo every 4 weeks for 24 weeks alongside continued treatment with hormone therapy.[17] There was a significant reduction in skeletal complications in the pamidronate group (56% versus 67%, P = 0.027) substantially reducing the skeletal morbidity from osteolytic metastases.

Results from the Danish cancer co-operative study in postmenopausal women with stage II or III breast cancer after mastectomy and limited axillary clearance suggest that tamoxifen combined with postoperative radiotherapy to chest wall and regional lymph nodes reduces the risk of locoregional recurrence (8% versus 35%), improves disease free survival (36% versus 24%) and overall survival (45% versus 36% at 10 years) when compared to tamoxifen alone.[18]

MELANOMA

SENTINEL NODE

In a study of 87 patients with early stage melanoma, Bostick[3] investigated the use of isosulfan blue dye combined with a radiopharmaceutical agent in the intra-operative detection of sentinel nodes. He concluded that the blue dye technique remains the criterion standard for sentinel node detection in melanoma, but that the addition of a radiopharmaceutical tracer serves as a useful adjunct. This was confirmed in the Multicentre Lymphadenectomy Trial; Morton et al.[19] have validated the accuracy of lymphatic mapping (LM) , sentinel lymphadenectomy (SL) and selective complete lymph node dissection in early stage melanoma. After a learning phase of 30 patients in each participating centre, results were compared with the organizing John Wayne Institute. In both centres, LM performed with blue dye plus radiocolloid was more successful (99.1%) than LM performed with blue dye alone (95.2%) ($P = 0.014$).They concluded that LM and SL can be successfully learned and applied in a standardized fashion with high accuracy by centres world-wide.

CHEMOTHERAPY

Several studies have investigated the incorporation of additional immuno and chemotherapeutic agents to current treatment regimens for metastatic melanoma.

Dorval et al.[20] evaluated the response rate, survival, and toxicity of treatment with cisplatin and high dose intravenous continuous infusion interleukin-2 (IL-2) with or without interferon-alpha-2a (IFN) in 117 patients with metastatic melanoma. The results indicated that the addition of IFN, in this trial, failed to significantly improve the activity of a cisplatin/IL-2 regimen in patients with metastatic melanoma.

Malignant melanoma metastasising to the brain is generally treated by radiotherapy as the blood brain barrier has proved a bar to conventional chemotherapy. In a trial of cisplatin and etoposide in the treatment of brain metastases, patients with breast and non-small cell lung cancer deposits showed some therapeutic response, 8 patients with melanoma showed no response to treatment.[21]

UPPER GI/HEPATOBILIARY

GALLBLADDER

Prophylactic antibiotics are frequently given prior to laparoscopic cholecystectomy. Higgins et al.[22] studied 450 patients given single i.v. dose of cefotetan, cephazolin or placebo. Ten postoperative infections were equally distributed throughout the three groups.

ANTI-REFLUX SURGERY

Chronic gastro-oesophageal reflux disease (GORD) is progressive in up to 25% of patients. Csendes et al.[23] have published the late results of a study of 164 patients with at least 3 years of symptomatic GORD. Between 1985 and 1997, patients were randomised to either fundoplication or calibration of the cardia. Overall recurrence at 5 years was ~20% and at 10 years ~40% for the two procedures. However, there was a significant difference in the recurrence rate between patients with and without Barretts oesophagus (45% versus 15% at 5 years and 83% versus 23% at 10 years after fundoplication and 57% versus 19% at 5 years and 80% versus 22% at 10 years after calibration). The authors conclude that anti-reflux procedures are effective in patients without Barretts, but that patients with Barretts should be considered for alternative surgical procedures or medical intervention.

Laparosopic Nissen fundoplication was compared to anterior partial fundoplication in a trial of 107 patients.[24] Control of reflux was similar in the two groups at 6 month follow-up. The anterior approach resulted in lower oesophageal sphincter pressures and less dysphagia.

ACHALASIA

Botulinum toxin has been studied in the treatment of achalasia and compared with pneumatic dilatation. Vaezi et al.[25] demonstrated a higher recurrence rate using toxin.

OESOPHAGEAL MALIGNANCY

Following randomisation to retrosternal or posterior mediastinal recon-struction, postoperative function and quality of life were assessed.[26] Retrosternal reconstruction showed an increased morbidity (15% versus 13%) and mortality (14.2% versus 8.3%) with higher retention of liquid and solid tracers in radionuclide transit studies. The posterior mediastinal route for reconstruction is to be recommended except in the face of incomplete resection.

Long-term follow-up results of 196 patients with locally advanced oesophageal malignancy demonstrated significantly better 5 year survival (26%) after chemoradiotherapy than after radiotherapy alone.[27]

GASTRIC MALIGNANCY

Controversy still exists over the optimal surgical resection for potentially curable gastric cancer. The MRC trial[28] randomized 400 patients to D1 (removal of regional perigastric nodes) or D2 (extended lymphadenectomy to include level 1 and 2 regional nodes) resection. 96% of patients have now been followed up for 3 years or to death, (median follow-up 6.5 years). The 5 year survival rates were 35% D1 and 33% D2. This trial does not support the Japanese experience of improved survival after more radical surgery.

Some 996 patients have been entered in the Dutch trial of D1 versus D2 resection.[29] They also report increased complications (43% in D2 versus 25% D1, $P = 0.001$), increased peri-operative death (10% D2 versus 4% D1, $P = 0.004$) with similar 5 year survival and do not recommend the routine use of D2 dissection for gastric cancer.

Despite the European findings, the Japanese are advocating a nation-wide study comparing D3 with D4 resection.[30]

In a trial of 618 patients with gastric malignancy over 6 cm from the cardia randomised to subtotal (SG) or total gastrectomy (TG) (both procedures included regional lymphadenectomy) 5-year survival was 65.3% SG versus 62.4% TG provided there was no intraperitoneal or distant spread.[31] SG is recommended as the procedure of choice.

The construction of a jejunal pouch after total gastrectomy was associated with slower emptying of the upper gut, improved eating capacity and fewer postoperative symptoms when compared to Roux-en-Y reconstruction in 49 patients studied by Jivonen.[32]

Locally advanced or metastatic gastric cancer not amenable to surgical resection may respond to chemotherapy (5-FU with epirubicin). In a study of 112 patients those treated with cisplatin in combination with 5-FU and epirubicin showed 42.6% versus 28.6% response rate and significant improvement in mean survival of 9.6 versus 7.1 months.[33]

PANCREATIC MALIGNANCY

One study compared the outcomes of Whipple's procedure with pylorus preserving pancreatoduodectomy (PPPD) in 31 patients.[34] There was no significant difference in outcome in terms of operative mortality, morbidity, operating time, blood loss or transfusion. PPPD was associated with more frequently delayed gastric emptying.

Opinions differ over the use of pancreatogastrostomy and pancreato-jejunostomy after PPPD; 23 patients randomised to either technique were reviewed for 2 years.[35] No differences in exocrine function, physical condition or pancreatic duct obstruction were detected.

Between 25–75% of patients with peri-ampullary carcinoma are found to be unresectable at operation and undergo biliary bypass. The question arises whether to perform prophylactic bypass to prevent late gastric outflow obstruction. In a study of 87 patients deemed not to be at significant risk of gastric outflow obstruction at the time of attempted pancreaticoduodenectomy, 44 underwent prophylactic retrocolic bypass and 43 did not.[36] There was no postoperative mortality and morbidity and postoperative stay were similar. Median survival was 8.3 months in both groups; however, 8/43 patients without bypass developed duodenal obstruction requiring intervention compared to none in the already bypassed group.

A more radical pancreaticoduodenectomy including distal gastrectomy and retroperitoneal lymphadenectomy was compared with standard pancreatico-duodenectomy (removing only the peripancreatic nodes en bloc with the specimen).[37] Of the 114 patients randomized, 56 patients underwent standard operation and 58 the radical procedure. There were no significant differences in the two groups comparing operative time, blood loss, morbidity (34%

versus 40%) and mortality (3 versus 2). One year actuarial survival was 77% for the standard group and 83% for the more radical group. Longer term results are awaited.

LIVER METASTASES

Several recently published randomised controlled trials have investigated alternative approaches to the management of colorectal liver metastases.

Intra-arterial chemotherapy

57 patients with unresectable colorectal metastases confined to the liver, and an indwelling catheter in the hepatic artery were included in a trial to compare two regimens of intra-arterial chemotherapy with 5-FU and folinic acid.[38] Median follow-up was 21 months, and estimated median survival 19 months; 29 patients (51%) have responded, 5 completely. Six patients experienced WHO grade 3 or 4 toxicity. There was no significant difference between the two regimens. Further results of this trial comparing intra-arterial infusion with conventional chemotherapy are awaited.

Intra-arterial adjuvant treatment after liver resection

Rudroff et al.[39] investigated the use of adjuvant intra-arterial chemotherapy (4 courses of mitomycin C and 5-FU) in 30 patients undergoing liver resection following surgery for Dukes C colorectal cancer between July 1984 to December 1985. In group-A (14 patients), an hepatic artery catheter was placed during liver resection; 16 group B control patients received no chemotherapy. After 5 years, 29% of patients were alive, but there was no significant difference in either 5 year survival or long term disease-free status between groups A and B. The initial tumour relapse was shifted towards extrahepatic sites in group A patients, but no difference was obtained regarding the definite distribution of recurrent disease.

Radiofrequency ablation

Curley et al.[40] treated 169 tumours in 123 patients with unresectable hepatic and metastatic malignancy using radiofrequency ablation (RFA) in a non-randomised trial to assess complications, treatment response, and recurrence of malignant disease. There were no treatment-related deaths, and the complication rate after RFA was 2.4%. All treated tumours were completely necrotic on imaging studies after completion of RFA treatments. With a median follow-up of 15 months, tumour has recurred in 3 of 169 treated lesions (1.8%), but metastatic disease has developed at other sites in 34 patients (27.6%). They concluded that RFA is a well tolerated and effective treatment for primary and secondary hepatic malignancy.

PRINGLE'S MANOEUVRE

Massive haemorrhage during liver resection remains a potentially lethal complication. Many surgeons employ Pringle's manoeuvre to reduce blood loss during resection; however, the upper limit of duration of this manoeuvre is not known. Man et al.[41] compared two groups of patients, those without use of the manoeuvre (n = 50) and those in which the lesser omentum was occluded with a clamp for repeated periods of 20 min with 5 min clamp free intervals (n = 62). Substantial liver damage as determined by liver function test and arterial ketone body ratio (AKBR) occurred after 120 min of accumulated clamp-time. Clamping for less than 120 min reduced blood loss, transfusion requirements and resection time resulting in rapid recovery of AKBR. Clamping for > 120 min had a significantly lower recovery rate of AKBR.

HEPATOCELLULAR CARCINOMA

Advanced unresectable hepatocellular carcinoma (HCC) has a median survival of less than 6 months. Gebbia et al.[42] have published the results of a phase II trial of 5-FU in modulation with intravenous high-dose levofolinic acid and oral hydroxyurea (HU) in a total of 50 consecutive patients none of whom had received previous chemotherapy. The median survival was 5.8 months (range 2.0–12.0+) The combination of 5-FU with levofolinic acid and oral HU on a weekly schedule was largely inactive against unresectable or metastatic HCC and results are no better than historical data reported for 5-FU alone.

A study comparing intra-arterial versus systemic administration of doxorubicin for non-resectable HCC showed no difference in survival (mean 7 versus 6.5 months).[43]

TRANSPLANT

The technique of ex vivo hepatic perfusion, first developed and used clinically in the 1970s by Abouna et al., has now been redesigned in a perfusion circuitry that mimics the physiological conditions of a normal liver.[44] Acute hepatic failure was induced in 18 dogs divided into three treatment groups. A control group (6 animals) received medical support, 12 animals were connected to the ex vivo liver support apparatus during acute hepatic failure via an AV shunt using a dog (n = 6) or calf liver (n = 6). All control animals died of progressive hepatic failure at 14–19 h after clamping the hepatic artery. The animals treated with ex vivo liver showed remarkable clinical and biochemical improvement. Five animals survived for 36–60 h. Another seven animals recovered completely and became long-term survivors with biochemical and histological evidence of regeneration of their own liver. These results strongly confirm that extracorporeal perfusion through a whole liver, using the system described, is possible for the treatment of acute, but reversible hepatic failure, as well as serving as a bridge to liver transplantation.

Corticosteroids are commonly used as immunosuppressants after liver transplantation. However, they are associated with considerable side-effects and recent work suggested that their routine use was unnecessary. The effects of early immunosuppression without the use of prednisolone were investigated in 45 patients randomized to receive no prednisolone or treatment for 3 months.[45] At a median follow-up of 14 months, survival in the two groups was not significantly different (70.2% versus 78.3%, P = 0.83), mild and moderate acute rejection were also similar.

Biliary reconstruction after transplantation has been the subject of much debate. Reconstruction in the absence of a T-tube is now accepted but disagreement over 'side-to-side' versus 'end-to-end' continues. Davidson et al.[46] studied 100 patients randomised to either reconstruction. Patients were followed up by ERCP at 2 weeks. After median follow-up of 53 months, there were no differences in biliary complications, leak rate or biliary stricture.

VARICEAL BLEEDING

Variceal bleeding is a major cause of mortality in patients with known portal hypertension (PHT). Conservative prevention of the first episode of variceal bleeding with propranolol is associated with side-effects, complicated by non-compliance and in some cases is not effective. Endoscopic variceal ligation (EVL) is now accepted as treatment for bleeding oesophageal varices. De et al.[47] randomised 30 cirrhotic patients with PHT, grades III and IV oesophageal varices, hepatic venous pressure gradient $\geq$ 12 mmHg and no prior history of upper gastrointestinal bleeding to receive propranolol (to reduce their pulse rate by 25% from baseline, $n = 15$) or EVL (weekly to fortnightly until variceal eradication, $n = 15$). All the patients in EVL group had variceal eradication during 3.8 ± 2.2 sessions. During a follow-up period of 17.6 ± 4.7 months, varices recurred in three patients treated with EVL, two of which bled (requiring further ligation). In contrast, during this period of follow-up one patient in the propranolol group had variceal bleeding; this difference was not significant.

The combination of variceal ligation with sclerotherapy has no benefit in the eradication of varices over ligation alone. A total of 60 patients undergoing weekly treatment until eradication was obtained were reviewed at 3 and 6 months. There was no difference in time to eradication, rebleeding, transfusion requirement or stricture formation.[48]

HYDATID DISEASE

Dziri et al.[49] recommend the use of omentoplasty after de-roofing or pericystectomy for hydatid disease of the liver. A total of 115 consecutive patients with single or multiloculated liver hydatid were randomly allocated to omentoplasty (OP) or not (NO) between January 1993 and December 1996. Main outcome measures included deep bleeding, haematoma, infection, or bile leakage. Secondary measures included wound complications, extra-abdominal complications, duration of operation, and length of hospital stay. Overall, there was a significant reduction in the incidence of deep intra-abdominal complications particularly abscesses in the group undergoing OP.

COLORECTAL

HAEMORRHOIDECTOMY

Two studies have compared stapled haemorrhoidectomy to diathermy excision haemorrhoidectomy. These include 62 patients randomly assigned to either treatment. Average pain in the stapled group was significantly reduced in both studies; the stapled patients also returned to normal activity earlier. Mehigan et al.[50] reported shorter anaesthetic time for the stapled group and

Rowsell et al.[51] reported shorter hospital stay. Early and late complications appear similar in both studies in the short term, longer term results are awaited.

Post haemorrhoidectomy pain remains a challenging problem. Transcutaneous electrical nerve stimulation (TENS) was administered to 30 patients after haemorrhoidectomy, pain scores 8, 12, 16 and 24 h postoperatively, analgesic use and postoperative complications were assessed.[52] TENS significantly reduced the requirement for opiates administered via patient controlled analgesic device (11.6 ± 2.2 mg for control group versus 6.2 ± 1.3 mg).

Day case haemorrhoidectomy was investigated by Carapeti et al.[53] in a study comparing open with closed technique. All 35 patients had healed within 6 weeks, there were no significant differences in pain score, analgesia requirement, return to normal activity or patient satisfaction scores.

Rubber band ligation of haemorrhoids is an effective out-patient treatment. Post ligation discomfort is not uncommon in ~25% of patients. Two studies investigated the use of lignocaine or bupivicaine injected into the ligated haemorrhoid tissue.[54,55] Neither had an effect on reducing pain in the long-term.

FISSURE IN ANO

The conservative treatment of anal fissures remains a fertile area. GTN is certainly effective but patients are troubled by its side-effects (mainly headaches). Research continues using agents which act to relax the smooth muscle complex.

Kennedy et al.[56] published the long-term results of a placebo controlled trial of GTN in the treatment of anal fissures in 43 patients. GTN reduced resting anal pressures and pain scores with a healing rate of 46% versus 16% in the placebo group (P = 0.001). Carapeti demonstrated healing rates of 67% compared to 32% for placebo (P = 0.008) but of those fissures that healed, 33% recurred.[57]

Topical nifedipine, acting through calcium channel blockade, was used to treat 283 patients.[58] At 21 days, 95% of fissures had healed compared to 50% of the placebo group (no treatment).

Brindisi et al.[59] also demonstrated 96% healing of chronic fissure using botulinum toxin compared with 60% healing in the GTN treated controls.

STAPLING DEVICES

Transanally inserted circular staplers have enabled the adoption of sphincter saving surgery, but the extent and nature of any damage to the sphincter complex is unknown. Fifty-eight consecutive patients with sigmoid adenocarcinoma were randomly assigned to transanally inserted stapler or biofragmentable anastomotic ring (avoiding anal manipulation) groups.[60] Anorectal manometry and clinical bowel function assessment were performed by an independent blinded observer before, 6 weeks and 6 months after surgery. At 6 weeks, there was significant impairment of mean anal resting pressures (mean impairment 23%, P <0.001) and physiological anal length (mean impairment 31%, P <0.01) in the stapled group. Pressures remained impaired at 6 months. Postoperative bowel function was no different between the two groups.

FAECAL INCONTINENCE

Faecal incontinence affects 2% of the adult population, rising to 7% in those over 65 years. External sphincter damage is often improved by surgical repair but internal sphincter injury is less amenable to surgical intervention. Phenylephrine is an α-adrenergic agonist which increases resting sphincter pressure in healthy volunteers. Carapeti et al.[61] investigated its topical use in the treatment of faecal incontinence secondary to internal sphincter dysfunction. They found no significant difference in incontinence score, resting anal pressure and anodermal blood flow between the phenylephrine and placebo treatment.

A total of 20 female patients with neurogenic faecal incontinence were studied in a trial comparing post anal repair, and total pelvic floor repair (post anal repair plus anterior levatorplasty and sphincter plication).[62] There was no significant difference between clinical, manometric, and radiological parameters measured before and 12 weeks after surgery in either group.

INFLAMMATORY BOWEL DISEASE

Sucralfate and methylprednisolone enemas are equally effective in the treatment of ulcerative proctosigmoiditis when administered twice daily and assessed clinically (by sigmoidoscopy) or histologically.[63]

Macroscopic recurrence of Crohn's disease occurs only weeks after 'curative' resection. Oral budesonide taken for one year and compared with a placebo in 88 patients showed only a small non-significant improvement in the endoscopic appearance, histological score and Crohn's disease activity index and cannot be recommended for prophylaxis in this setting.[64]

PREVENTION AND SCREENING FOR MALIGNANCY

A putative approach to the chemoprevention of colonic cancer is the use of nutrients or drugs to modify altered growth and differentiation of mucosal cells towards normal.

Forty patients, ages 25–79 years, with a history of a large bowel adenoma or a first-degree relative with large bowel cancer were randomised in a cross-over trial to test the effects of high (6 dairy servings/day) or low dairy intake (< 0.5 serving of dairy products/day), diets on rectal mucosal proliferation.[65] There was no statistically significant change in rectal mucosal cell proliferation (estimated by immunohistochemical determination of proliferating cell nuclear antigen and whole crypt mitotic count).

However, increasing the daily intake of calcium via low-fat dairy food in 70 subjects with a history of polypectomy for colonic adenomatous polyps randomized to 4 strata by diet (control versus higher calcium up to 1200 mg/day) and age (< 60 versus ≥ 60 years) reduced proliferative activity of colonic epithelial cells and restored the markers of cellular differentiation.[66] During 6 and 12 months of treatment, reduction of colonic epithelial cell proliferative activity ($P < 0.05$), reduction in size of the proliferative compartment ($P < 0.05$), and restoration of acidic mucin ($P < 0.02$), cytokeratin AE1 distribution ($P < 0.05$), and nuclear size ($P < 0.05$) toward that of normal cells occurred. Control subjects showed no differences from baseline proliferative values at 6 and 12 months ($P > 0.05$).

Four year follow-up results of the Nottingham trial of faecal occult blood screening in a population of 150,000 have shown improved survival in patients with screen detected cancers.[67]

RECTAL CARCINOMA

The Swedish Rectal Cancer Trial has unequivocally demonstrated that pre-operative high-dose (5 x 5 Gy) radiotherapy reduces local recurrence rates and improves overall survival. Of the original 220 patients included in the Swedish trial, 171 completed a questionnaire investigating the effect of pre-operative high-dose radiotherapy on long-term bowel function following anterior resection.[68] Median bowel frequency per week was 20 in the irradiated group ($n = 84$) and 10 in the surgery-alone group ($n = 87$; $P <0.001$). Incontinence for loose stools ($P <0.001$), urgency ($P <0.001$), and emptying difficulties ($P <0.05$) were all more common after irradiation. Of the irradiated group, 30% stated that they had an impaired social life because of bowel dysfunction, compared with 10% of the surgery-alone group ($P <0.01$). This emphasizes the need to identify predictive factors for local recurrence to allow selection of patients with high probability of cure with surgery alone.

Herrmann et al.[69] published the late results of a trial comparing pre-operative radiotherapy with selective postoperative radiotherapy; 94 patients with operable carcinoma of the rectum were included. Of these, 47 patients were treated 24–48 h prior to surgery with 5 x 3.3 Gy and 46 patients received no preoperative treatment. Patients in either group received postoperative irradiation if risk factors (T4-stage, R1/R2 resection, intra-operative tumour perforation) were present. Total post-operative doses of 41.4 Gy (pre-operative irradiation) or 59.8 Gy (surgery only) were applied with doses per fraction of 1.8–2.0 Gy. Pre-operative irradiation significantly reduced the incidence of local recurrence in R0-resected patients (24% versus 13%, $P = 0.08$). The time to recurrence was delayed (1.9 versus 3 years). The 5-year actuarial survival rate was significantly higher in the pre-operatively irradiated group compared to the not pre-irradiated group (40% versus 28%, $P = 0.027$).

Postoperative chemotherapy with radiotherapy is known to improve survival in rectal tumours. The addition of the 5-FU modulator leucovorin was investigated in a trial of 220 patients randomized postoperatively to receive radiotherapy with 5-FU and leucovorin versus radiotherapy and 5-FU.[70] After median follow up of 4.9 years, no significant difference in disease-free survival was demonstrated. Severe toxicity was associated with the use of leucovorin.

Voiding dysfunction is frequently observed after rectal resection and justifies urinary drainage. Benoist et al.[71] compared 1 versus 5 days of transurethral catheterisation after rectal resection. The acute urinary retention rate was comparable in the two groups but the urinary tract infection rate was significantly lower in the 1-day group versus the 5-day group (14% versus 40%, $P <0.01$).

PELVIC DRAINAGE

Anastomotic leakage after colorectal resection is more prevalent when the anastomosis is infraperitoneal. The benefit of pelvic drainage has been questioned. A total of 494 patients (249 men and 245 women), mean age 66 ± 15 years (range 15–101 years), with any disorder located from the right colon to the midrectum undergoing resection followed by rectal or anal anastomosis were randomized to undergo either drainage (n = 248) with 2 multiperforated 14F suction drains or no drainage (n = 246). The overall leakage rate was 6.3% with no significant difference between those with or without drainage. The rate of other intra-abdominal and extra-abdominal complications did not differ significantly between the 2 groups.

These findings were supported by the systematic review of previously published papers comparing the effects of pelvic drainage with no drainage. Concluding that the use of a drain did not significantly affect mortality, clinical and radiological anastomotic leakage rate, wound infection rate, or major complication rate.[72]

References

1. The MRC Laparoscopic Groin Hernia Trial Group. Laparoscopic versus open repair of groin hernia: a randomised comparison. Lancet 1999; 354: 185–190.
2. Picchio M, Lombardi A, Zolovkins A, Mihelsons M, La Torre G. Tension-free laparoscopic and open hernia repair: randomized controlled trial of early results. World J Surg 1999; 23: 1004–1007; discussion 1008–1009.
3. Johansson B, Hallerback B, Glise H, Anesten B, Smedberg S, Roman J. Laparoscopic mesh versus open preperitoneal mesh versus conventional technique for inguinal hernia repair: a randomized multicenter trial (SCUR Hernia Repair Study). Ann Surg 1999; 230: 225–231.
4. Juul P, Christensen K. Randomized clinical trial of laparoscopic versus open inguinal hernia repair. Br J Surg 1999; 86: 316–319.
5. Danielsson P, Isacson S, Hansen MV. Randomized study of Lichtenstein compared with Shouldice inguinal hernia repair by surgeons in training. Eur J Surg 1999; 165: 49–53.
6. Fuhii Y, Tanaka H, Kawasaki T. Randomized clinical trial of granisetron, droperidol and metoclopramide for the treatment of nausea and vomiting after laparoscopic cholecystectomy. Br J Surg 2000; 87: 285–288.
7. Underwood RA, Dunnegan DL, Soper NJ. Prospective, randomized trial of bipolar electrosurgery versus ultrasonic coagulation for division of short gastric vessels during laparoscopic Nissen fundoplication. Surg Endosc 1999; 13: 763–768.
8. Hebert PC, Wells G, Blajchman MA, Marshall J, Martin C, Pagliarello G. A multicenter randomized controlled clinical trial of transfusion requirements in critical care. N Engl J Med 1999; 340: 409–417.
9. Alexander FE, Anderson TJ, Brown HK, Forrest APM, Hepburn W, Kirkpatrick AE. 14 years of follow-up from the Edinburgh randomised trial of breast-cancer screening. Lancet 1999; 353: 1903–1908.
10. Cummings SR, Eckert S, Krueger KA et al. The effect of raloxifene on risk of breast cancer in postmenopausal women: results from the MORE randomized trial. Multiple outcomes of raloxifene evaluation. JAMA 1999; 281: 2189–2197.
11. Thomas R, Alvino P, Cortino GR et al. Long-acting versus short-acting cephalosporins for preoperative prophylaxis in breast surgery: a randomized double-blind trial involving 1,766 patients. Chemotherapy 1999; 45: 217–223.
12. Hata Y, Uchino J, Asaishi K et al. UFT and mitomycin plus tamoxifen for stage II, ER-positive breast cancer. Hokkaido ACETBC Study Group. Oncology 1999; 13 (Suppl. 3): 91–95.
13. Vrieling C, Collette L, Fourquet A et al. The influence of the boost in breast-conserving therapy on cosmetic outcome in the EORTC "boost versus no boost" trial. EORTC Radiotherapy and Breast Cancer Cooperative Groups. European Organization for Research and Treatment of Cancer. Int J Radiat Oncol Biol Physics 1999; 45: 677–685.

14. Hardenbergh PH, Recht A, Gollamudi S et al. Treatment-related toxicity from a randomized trial of the sequencing of doxorubicin and radiation therapy in patients treated for early stage breast cancer. Int J Radiat Oncol Biol Physics 1999; 45: 69–72.

15. Mauriac L, Durand M, Avril A, Dilhuydy JM. Effects of primary chemotherapy in conservative treatment of breast cancer patients with operable tumors larger tha 3 cm. Results of a randomized trial in a single centre. Ann Oncol 1991; 2: 347–354.

16. Harper-Wynne C, English J, Meyer L et al. Randomized trial to compare the efficacy and toxicity of cyclophosphamide, methotrexate and 5-fluorouracil (CMF) with methotrexate mitoxantrone (MM) in advanced carcinoma of the breast. Br J Cancer 1999; 81: 316–322.

17. Theirault RL, Lipton A, Hortobagyi GN et al. Pamidronate reduces skeletal morbidity in women with advanced breast cancer and lytic bone lesions: a randomized, placebo-controlled trial. Protocol 18 Aredia Breast Cancer Study Group. J Clin Oncol 1999; 17: 846–854.

18. Overgaard M, Jensen MB, Overgaard J et al. Postoperative radiotherapy in high-risk postmenopausal breast-cancer patients given adjuvant tamoxifen: Danish Breast Cancer Cooperative Group DBCG 82c trial. Lancet 1999; 353: 1641–1648.

19. Morton DL, Thompson JF, Essner R et al. Validation of the accuracy of intraoperative lymphatic mapping and sentinel lymphadenectomy for early-stage melanoma: a multicenter trial. Multicenter Selective Lymphadenectomy Trial Group. Ann Surg 1999; 230: 453–465.

20. Dorval T, Negrier S, Chevreau C et al. Randomized trial of treatment with cisplatin and interleukin-2 either alone or in combination with interferon-alpha-2a in patients with metastatic melanoma: a Federation Nationale des Centres de Lutte Contre le Cancer Multicenter, parallel study. Cancer 1999; 85: 1060–1066.

21. Franciosi V, Cocconi G, Michiara M et al. Front-line chemotherapy with cisplatin and etoposide for patients with brain metastases from breast carcinoma, nonsmall cell lung carcinoma, or malignant melanoma: a prospective study. Cancer 1999; 85: 1599–1605.

22. Higgins A, London J, Charland S, Ratzer E, Clark J, Haun W. Prophylactic antibiotics for elective laparoscopic cholecystectomy: are they necessary? Arch Surg 1999; 134: 611–614.

23. Csendes A, Burdiles P, Korn O, Braghetto I, Huertas C, Rojas J. Late results of a randomized clinical trial comparing total fundoplication versus calibration of the cardia with posterior gastropexy. Br J Surg 2000; 87: 289–297.

24. Watson DI, Jamieson GG, Pike GK, Davies N, Richardson M, Devitt PG. Prospective randomized double-blind trial between laparoscopic Nissen fundoplication and anterior partial fundoplication. Br J Surg 1999; 86: 123–130.

25. Vaezi MF, Richter JE, Wilcox CM, Schroeder PL, Birgisson S, Slaughter RL. Botulinum toxin versus pneumatic dilatation in the treatment of achalasia: a randomised trial. Gut 1999; 44: 231–239.

26. Gawad KA, Hosch SB, Bumann D et al. How important is the route of reconstruction after esophagectomy: a prospective randomized study. American Journal of Gastroenterology 1999; 94: 1490–1496.

27. Cooper JS, Gou MD, Herskovic A, Macdonald JS, Martenson JAJ, Al-Sarraf M. Chemoradiotherapy of locally advanced esophageal cancer: long term follow-up of prospective randomized trial. JAMA 1999; 281: 1623–1627.

28. Cuschieri A, Weeden S, Fielding J et al. Patient survival after D1 and D2 resections for gastric cancer: long-term results of the MRC randomized surgical trial. Surgical Co-operative Group. Br J Cancer 1999; 79: 1522–1530.

29. Bonenkamp JJ, Hermans J, Sasako M, van de Velde CJ. Extended lymph-node dissection for gastric cancer. Dutch Gastric Cancer Group [see comments]. N Engl J Med 1999; 340: 908–914.

30. Maeta M, Yamashiro H, Saito H et al. A prospective pilot study of extended (D3) and superextended para-aortic lymphadenectomy (D4) in patients with T3 or T4 gastric cancer managed by total gastrectomy. Surgery 1999; 125: 325–331.

31. Bozzetti F, Marubini E, Bonfanti G, Miceli R, Piano C, Gennari L. Subtotal versus total gastrectomy for gastric cancer: five-year survival rates in a multicenter randomized Italian trial. Italian Gastrointestinal Tumor Study Group. Ann Surg 1999; 230: 170–178.

32. Jivonen MK, Koskinen MO, Ikonen TJ, Matikainen MJ. Emptying of the jejunal pouch and Roux-en-Y limb after total gastrectomy – a randomised prospective study. Eur J Surg 1999; 165: 742–747.

33. Roth A, Kolaric K, Zupanc D, Oresic V, Ebling Z. High doses of 5-fluorouracil and epirubicin with or without cisplatin in advanced gastric cancer: a randomized study. Tumori 1999; 85: 234–238.

34. Lin PW, Lin YJ. Prospective randomized comparison between pylorus-preserving and standard pancreaticoduodenectomy. Br J Surg 1999; 86: 603–607.

35. Konishi M, Ryu M, Kinoshita T, Inoue K. Pathophysiology after pylorus-preserving pancreatoduodenectomy: a comparative study of pancreatogastrostomy and pancreatojejunostomy. Hepatogastroenterology 1999; 46: 1181–1186.

36. Lillemoe KD, Cameron JL, Hardacre JM et al. Is prophylactic gastrojejunostomy indicated for unresectable periampullary cancer? A prospective randomized trial. Ann Surg 1999; 230: 322–330.

37. Yeo CJ, Cameron JL, Sohn TA et al. Pancreaticoduodenectomy with or without extended retroperitoneal lymphadenectomy for periampullary adenocarcinoma: comparison of morbidity and mortality and short-term outcome. Ann Surg 1999; 229: 613–624.

38. Howell JD, Warren HW, Anderson JH, Kerr DJ, McArdle CS. Intra-arterial 5-fluorouracil and intravenous folinic acid in the treatment of liver metastases from colorectal cancer. Eur J Surg 1999; 165: 652–658.

39. Rudroff C, Altendorf-Hoffmann A, Stangl R, Scheele J. Prospective randomised trial on adjuvant hepatic-artery infusion chemotherapy after R0 resection of colorectal liver metastases. Langenbecks Arch Surg 1999; 384: 243–249.

40. Curley SA, Izzo F, Delrio P et al. Radiofrequency ablation of unresectable primary and metastatic hepatic malignancies: results in 123 patients [see comments]. Ann Surg 1999; 230: 1–8.

41. Man K, Fan ST, Ng IO et al. Tolerance of the liver to intermittent Pringle maneuver in hepatectomy for liver tumors. Arch Surg 1999; 134: 533–539.

42. Gebbia V, Maiello E, Serravezza G et al. 5-Fluorouracil plus high dose levofolinic acid and oral hydroxyurea for the treatment of primary hepatocellular carcinomas: results of a phase II multicenter study of the Southern Italy Oncology Group (GOIM). Anticancer Res 1999; 19: 1407–1410.

43. Tzoracoleftherakis EE, Spiliotis JD, Kyriakopoulou T, Kakkos SK. Intra-arterial versus systemic chemotherapy for non-operable hepatocellular carcinoma. Hepatogastroenterology 1999; 46: 1122–1125.

44. Abouna GM, Ganguly PK, Hamdy HM, Jabur SS, Tweed WA, Costa G. Extracorporeal liver perfusion system for successful hepatic support pending liver regeneration or liver transplantation: a pre-clinical controlled trial. Transplantation 1999; 67: 1576–1583.

45. Tisone G, Angelico M, Palmieri G et al. A pilot study on the safety and effectiveness of immunosuppression without prednisone after liver transplantation. Transplantation 1999; 67: 1308–1313.

46. Davidson BR, Rai R, Kurzawinski TR, Selves L, Farouk M, Dooley J. Prospective randomized trial of end-to-end versus side-to-side biliary reconstruciton after orthotopic liver transplantation. Br J Surg 1999; 86: 447–452.

47. De BK, Ghoshal UC, Das T, Santra A, Biswas PK. Endoscopic variceal ligation for primary prophylaxis of oesophageal variceal bleed: preliminary report of a randomized controlled trial. J Gastroenterol Hepatol 1999; 14: 220–224.

48. Al Traif I, Fachartz FS, Al Jumah A et al. Randomized trial of ligation versus combined ligation and sclerotherapy for bleeding esophageal varices [see comment]. Gastrointest Endosc 1999; 50: 1–6.

49. Dziri C, Paquet JC, Hay JM et al. Omentoplasty in the prevention of deep abdominal complications after surgery for hydatid disease of the liver: a multicenter, prospective, randomized trial. French Associations for Surgical Research. J Am Coll Surg 1999; 188: 281–289.

50. Mehigan BJ, Monson JRT, Hartley JE. Stapling procedure for haemorrhoids versus Milligan-Morgan haemorrhoidectomy: randomised controlled trial. Lancet 2000; 335: 782–785.

51. Rowsell M, Bello M, Hemingway DM. Circumferential mucosectomy (stapled haemorrhoidectomy) versus conventional haemorrhoidectomy: randomised controlled trial. Lancet 2000; 335: 779–781.

52. Chiu JH, Chen WS, Chen CH et al. Effect of transcutaneous electrical nerve stimulation

Recent randomised controlled trials in general surgery

for pain relief on patients undergoing hemorrhoidectomy: prospective, randomized, controlled trial. Dis Colon Rectum 1999; 42: 180–185.

53. Carapeti EA, Kamm MA, McDonald P, Chadwick SJD, Phillips RKS. Randomized trial of open versus closed day-case haemorrhoidectomy. Br J Surg 1999; 86: 612–613.

54. Law WL, Chu KW. Triple rubber band ligation for hemorrhoids: prospective, randomized trial of use of local anesthetic injection. Dis Colon Rectum 1999; 42: 363–366.

55. Hooker GD, Plewes EA, Rajgopal C, Taylor BM. Local injection of bupivacaine after rubber band ligation of hemorrhoids: prospective, randomized study. Dis Colon Rectum 1999; 42: 174–179.

56. Kennedy ML, Sowter S, Nguyen H, Lubowski DZ. Glyceryl trinitrate ointment for the treatment of chronic anal fissure: results of a placebo-controlled trial and long-term follow-up. Dis Colon Rectum 1999; 42: 1000–1006.

57. Carapeti EA, Kamm MA, McDonald PJ, Chadwick D, Melville D, Phillips RKS. Randomised controlled trial shows that glyceryl trinitrate heals anal fissures, higher doses are not more effective and there is a high recurrence rate. Gut 1999; 44: 727–730.

58. Antropoli C, Perrotti P, Rubino M, DeStefona G, Migliore G. Nifedipine for local use in conservative treatment of anal fissures: preliminary results of a multicenter study. Dis Colon Rectum 1999; 42: 1011–1015.

59. Brisinda D, Maria G, Bentivoglio AR, Cassetta E, Gui D, Albanese A. A comparison of injections of botulinim toxin and topical nitroglycerin ointment for the treatment of chronic anal fissure. N Engl J Med 1999; 341: 65–69.

60. Ho YH, Tan M, Leong A, Eu KW, Nyam D, Seow-Choen F. Anal pressures impaired by stapler insertion during colorectal anastomosis: a randomized, controlled trial. Dis Colon Rectum 1999; 42: 89–95.

61. Carapeti EA, Kamm MA, Phillips RKS. Randomized controlled trial of topical phenylephrine in the treatment of faecal incontinence. Br J Surg 2000; 87: 38–42.

62. van Tets WF, Kuijpers JH. Pelvic floor procedures produce no consistent changes in anatomy or physiology. Dis Colon Rectum 1998; 41: 365–369.

63. Wright JP, Winter TA, Candy S, Marks IS. Sucralfate and methylprednisolone enemas in active ulcerative colitis: a prospective, single-blind study. Dig Dis Sci 1999; 44: 1899–1901.

64. Ewe K, Bottger T, Buhr HJ, Ecker KW, Otto HF. Low-dose budesonide treatment for prevention of postoperative recurrence of Crohn's disease: a multicentre randomized placebo-controlled trial. German Budesonide Study Group. Eur J Gastroenterol Hepatol 1999; 11: 277–282.

65. Karagas MR, Tosteson TD, Greenberg ER et al. Effects of milk and milk products on rectal mucosal cell proliferation in humans. Cancer Epidemiol Biomarkers Prev 1998; 7: 757–766.

66. Holt PR, Atillasoy EO, Gilman J et al. Modulation of abnormal colonic epithelial cell proliferation and differentiation by low-fat dairy foods: a randomized controlled trial [see comments]. JAMA 1998; 280: 1074–1079.

67. Mapp tJ, Hardcastle JD, Moss SM, Robinson MHE. Survival of patients with colorectal cancer diagnosed in a randomized controlled trial of faecal occult blood screening. Br J Surg 1999; 86: 1286–1291.

68. Dahlberg M, Glimelius B, Graf W, Pahlman L. Preoperative irradiation affects functional results after surgery for rectal cancer: results from a randomized study. Dis Colon Rectum 1998; 41: 543–551.

69. Herrmann T, Petersen S, Hellmich G, Baumann M, Ludwig K. Delayed toxicity of brief preoperative irradiation and risk-adjusted postoperative radiotherapy of operative rectal carcinoma. Results of a randomized prospective study [in German]. Strahlentherap Onkol 1999; 175: 430–436.

70. Fountzilas G, Zisiadis A, Dafni U et al. Postoperative radiation and concomitant bolus fluorouracil with or without additional chemotherapy with fluorouracil and high-dose leucovorin in patients with high-risk rectal cancer: a randomized phase III study conducted by the Hellenic Cooperative Oncology Group. Ann Oncol 1999; 10: 671–676.

71. Benoist S, Panis Y, Denet C, Mauvais F, Mariani P, Valleur P. Optimal duration of urinary drainage after rectal resection: a randomized controlled trial. Surgery 1999; 125: 135–141.

72. Urbach DR, Kennedy ED, Cohen MM. Colon and rectal anastomoses do not require routine drainage: a systematic review and meta-analysis. Ann Surg 1999; 229: 174–180.

Index